Praise for *The Sabbath World*

"This hybrid of a book—part spiritual memoir, part religious history and sociological analysis and literary exegesis and philosophical musing—[is] a book of richness and depth. . . . Both riveting and moving."   —*The New York Times Book Review*

"Enormously interesting . . . Shulevitz, a gifted essayist, is the kind of writer who wears her erudition lightly."   —*The New Republic*

"A beautifully written, consistently engaging reflection on what [Shulevitz] calls 'the social morality of time' . . . This extended essay on commitment and discipline in our use of time will reward readers from any religious tradition. . . . *The Sabbath World* will stimulate your thinking about how to fill our unchanging need for discipline, ritual, household traditions, and committed study."
                                                            —*Commonweal*

"Judith Shulevitz's *The Sabbath World* is possibly the best popular work on the Sabbath since Heschel's immortal *The Sabbath* (1951). . . . Shulevitz writes elegant prose, and entwines her excellent discourse on the history, nature, and value of the Sabbath with her own story of struggle with Sabbath observance. . . . There is nobody who should not read this book."   —*Jewish Book World*

"You might think we've had enough books on this topic in recent years, but you'd be wrong, as evidenced by Judith Shulevitz's *The*

Sabbath World: Glimpses of a Different Order of Time, every chapter of which is a wise and winsome meditation on yet another aspect of this inexhaustible topic. . . . Shulevitz asks all the right questions."

—*Books & Culture: A Christian Review*

"This book is about longing—for home, holiness, ritual, love, food, drink, socializing, contemplating, above all longing for time to experience this fullness. . . . It's an intense book and intensely engaging, one that as a reader I didn't want to end." —*Chicago Tribune*

"Exceptionally illuminating." —*Haaretz Daily Newspaper*

"Wonderful . . . part of a small set of books that have helped me situate myself as a Jew and as a person."

—Jeffrey Goldberg, *The Atlantic*

"Judith Shulevitz has achieved something nearly impossible. She has written a book about the Sabbath that is truly singular. In fact, *The Sabbath World* could well become the Heschel-equivalent for a postmodern generation straining to hold on to the Sabbath against the allures of 24–7 technology and ecumenical politesse."

—*Moment* magazine

"Intellectually invigorating . . . [Readers will] be rewarded by Shulevitz's many engaging reflections on time, including its history, divisions and ethics, making reading this book a bracing, often illuminating experience." —*The New Leader*

THE SABBATH WORLD

THE
SABBATH
WORLD

GLIMPSES OF A
DIFFERENT ORDER OF TIME

JUDITH SHULEVITZ

RANDOM HOUSE TRADE PAPERBACKS / NEW YORK

2011 Random House Trade Paperback Edition

Copyright © 2010 by Judith Shulevitz
Reading group guide copyright © 2011 by Random House, Inc.

All rights reserved.

Published in the United States by Random House Trade Paperbacks,
an imprint of The Random House Publishing Group,
a division of Random House, Inc., New York.

RANDOM HOUSE TRADE PAPERBACKS and colophon are trademarks
of Random House, Inc.

Portions of this work were originally published in *The New York Times Magazine.*

Originally published in hardcover in the United States by Random House,
an imprint of The Random House Publishing Group,
a division of Random House, Inc., in 2010.

Library of Congress Cataloging-in-Publication Data
Shulevitz, Judith.
The Sabbath world : glimpses of a different order of time / Judith Shulevitz.
p.   cm.
Includes bibliographical references and index.
ISBN 978-0-8129-7173-6
1. Sabbath.   2. Sunday.   3. Time—Religious aspects—Judaism.   4. Time—
Religious aspects—Christianity.   5. Time—Psychological aspects.   6. Rest—
Religious aspects—Judaism.   7. Rest—Religious aspects—Christianity.
8. Shulevitz, Judith.   I. Title.
BM685.S478 2010
296.4'1—dc22   2009026417

Printed in the United States of America

www.atrandom.com

2 4 6 8 9 7 5 3 1

Book design by Susan Turner

To my mother

There was some puzzling, tormenting residue of the Sunday world within her, some persistent Sunday self, which insisted upon a relationship with the now shed-away vision world. How could one keep up a relationship with that which one denied?

D. H. LAWRENCE, *The Rainbow*

Whether I see it scattered down among tangled woods, or beaming broad across the fields, or hemmed in between brick buildings, or tracing out the figure of the casement on my chamber floor, still I recognize the Sabbath sunshine.—And ever let me recognize it! Some illusions, and this among them, are the shadows of great truths.

NATHANIEL HAWTHORNE, *Sunday at Home*

CONTENTS

INTRODUCTION

THE VIEW FROM AFAR

<u>1.</u>

AT SOME POINT WE ALL LOOK FOR A SABBATH, WHETHER OR NOT THAT'S what we call it. Organized religion need not be involved. As a child upset about having been moved from a house with a garden in a suburb of Detroit to a cramped apartment in downtown San Juan, Puerto Rico, I curled up in the space between a file cabinet and a freezer early on Saturday mornings. Not the freezer on top of the refrigerator in our kitchen but the full-size appliance my mother had put in a corner of our small sunroom. She had bought it to store the kosher meat she got flown in from the mainland every few months—there were no kosher butchers in San Juan. The Sabbath not being a day for taking meat out of the freezer, I didn't have to worry about my mother coming in. Nestled among thick electrical cords, I hugged my legs, rested my head and ribs against the metal side, and let the vibrations lull me into a prayerful self-pity. This was *my* Sabbath, hidden inside hers.

My mother went to the synagogue later that day, taking us children with her. The Conservative synagogue in San Juan, unlike the thriving Reform one across the street, seemed reserved for the aged and infirm—refugees from Batista's Cuba, some of them also refugees from what people were just starting to call the Holocaust. These old men and occasional women smelled funny, and sang funny, too. My siblings and I referred to one of them as "the foghorn." The building, a ruined mansion starting to crumble, smelled of wood rot. It had termites. The specks of wood they had chewed and shat out would fall from the tops of the prayer books in a fine spray of golden dust when you pulled them off their shelves.

Almost nothing is as hard to empathize with as the words and things that other people find comforting, especially when they seek that comfort in squalid surroundings. Seen from the outside, the quest for religious solace looks preposterous. Søren Kierkegaard said that religion has a truth so purely interior that it approaches madness. The encounter with the holy has been described as a flash of hidden knowledge, a suspicion, an awe, an elation, a dread, a mystery, a *mysterium tremendum*. Whatever it is, it requires a courage that is as much social as spiritual. The state associated with holiness "is perfectly *sui generis* and irreducible to any other," the theologian Rudolf Otto wrote in *The Idea of the Holy*. Insofar as it is untranslatable, the holy, not to mention the search for it, has the powerful potential to be lonely.

Why associate the Sabbath with solitude? By common consensus, the day is all about getting connected. It's the ancient equivalent of social-networking software. With its laws proscribing work and mandating social encounters—meals, gatherings, study sessions—the Sabbath blocks out time for shedding one's professional or workaday identity and weaving the bonds of a collective identity. All this is true. Yet at the core of the Sabbath lies an unassuageable longing. The Sabbath grasps after something that is out of reach. *Qadosh,* the Hebrew word for "holy," comes from a root that means "apart, separate, withdrawn." In Judaism, that which is holy is that which has been fenced off. The Sabbath rituals create this boundary, and the boundary creates the experience of otherness that we call the holy. But the inverse of this process is a yearning for an impossible ideal, a utopia that is by definition unattainable. The Law, the legal theorist Robert Cover says, is a bridge between our imperfect world and the vision of its perfection. Religious laws and rituals remind us that we live in exile, not in perfect harmony, neither with one another nor with God. Had my mother come upon me, she would have seen a troubled child in a dusty corner, not a girl using a freezer full of steak as her personal altar to the Midwest. When I entered that synagogue, I had no idea what my mother saw in it.

What *did* she see in it? I've never asked her, because she couldn't have told me what I wanted to know. How do you single out precisely which aspect of the Sabbath mitigates your particular loneliness? The setting, the rites, the prayer book—the Sabbath dramaturgy mixes them all up. Each element of the Jewish Sabbath bears traces of every period in which Jews kept it, which is every period in Jewish history. At any given moment, several different movies about the Sabbath will be playing simultaneously inside the head of the Sabbath observer. "Holy days, rituals, liturgies—all are like musical notations which, in themselves, cannot convey the nuances and textures of live performance," the historian Yosef Hayim Yerushalmi writes.

You might as well ask, What did God see on his Sabbath? There is an answer to that, believe it or not. It's angels, created by God so that *his* Sabbaths wouldn't be lonely, as they were before he gave the Sabbath to the Jews so that they would keep it with him. These angels are stock figures in the vast body of legends that has grown up around the Sabbath. They can be found in a retelling of the story of Creation in the book of Jubilees, written two hundred years before Christ was born, and in a hymnal found among the Dead Sea Scrolls called "Songs for the Sabbath Sacrifice," compiled a century later by the Essenes, a desert sect awaiting the end of the world. In the songs, the angels collect themselves on the Sabbath into a heavenly choir. When worshippers joined their voices to those of the angels, the two choruses formed a sort of otherworldly conference call, connecting the earthly and the divine.

In the centuries that followed, the rabbinic sages—teachers and consolers of a people nearly exterminated, then enslaved and scattered, after Judea's revolt against Roman rule in the second century C.E.—concocted myths about the Sabbath in which the Sabbath figured as *their* saving angel, their rescue from God's abandonment.

The Sabbath, said the rabbis, is a bride given by God to her groom, the people of Israel. Once a week, they go forth in wedding clothes to marry her.

The Sabbath, said the rabbis, is a gift from God's treasury. Once a week, his people receive it and are enriched.

The Sabbath, said the rabbis, is the Temple in time rather than space. Once a week, every Jew becomes a priest and enters it.

The Sabbath, said the rabbis, is the Chosen Day, just as the children of Israel are the Chosen People.

My favorite story makes the Sabbath a place in space rather than a point in time. "How do you know that Saturday is the Sabbath?" a Roman governor named Tinius Rufus is said to have asked the great sage Akiva in the second century. "Because of the river Sambatyon," Rabbi Akiva says. For it "carries stones the whole week but allows them to rest on the Sabbath," by which Akiva meant that six days a week the current of the Sambatyon is so strong that it pushes boulders along, but on the seventh it stops flowing entirely.

Akiva was not making this up, exactly. Other ancient writers—Greek as well as Jewish, Pliny the Elder and Josephus among them—also spoke of this magical river, though they put it in different places: Persia, Lebanon, Ethiopia. Six centuries later, Eldad the Danite, a dark-skinned Jew, appeared out of nowhere in a town called Kairouan in North Africa (now Tunisia), claiming to have been shipwrecked and captured by cannibals, and told a tale of the Sambatyon. Delivered in a Hebrew peppered with Arabisms, Eldad's stories had such a powerful effect on his audience that the elders of the town grew alarmed and wrote to the exilarch in Babylon, a princely figure who ruled over all Jews living in exile, asking for advice. The exilarch wrote back to the Jews of Kairouan saying that Eldad may have been telling the truth, since there were enough references to the ten lost tribes and the Sambatyon in rabbinic texts to back him up.

On the far side of the Sambatyon, said Eldad, live the sons of Moses, carried there by God when the Jews were marched away from Israel as slaves to the Babylonians in the sixth century B.C.E. Protected by God's cloud and by the sea, unable to cross their Sabbath-keeping river (since it's fordable only on the Sabbath and they, of course, keep the Sabbath, too), the sons of Moses dwell in perfect isolation and holiness. They occupy mansions and castles miraculously free of flies, lice, scorpions, and other swarming creatures deemed unclean by the Bible. They raise sheep, oxen, and chickens that give birth twice a year; tend to gardens of olives, pomegranates, figs, and melons that bear fruit just as often; speak Hebrew; take ritual baths; never swear; live to the age of a hundred or a hundred and twenty; and do all their own chores, "for they have no manservants or maidservants, and they are all equal."

Tinius Rufus didn't ask Rabbi Akiva where this phantasmagorical Sabbatical river had its source. But Akiva might have had an answer. The rabbis tell us that it flows from a spring in Paradise. That is the detail that breaks my heart. For, unlike the bride of the Sabbath and the gift of the Sabbath, the river of the Sabbath lies forever hidden from view, offering ordinary humans neither the longed-for transport nor relief. That the Sambatyon partakes of earthly geography suggests that God is present in his creation, but that the river has its source in Paradise hints darkly that he can never be reached.

In any event, Akiva did not convert Tinius Rufus to Judaism (though some rabbinic legends have him converting Tinius Rufus's wife). This interfaith dialogue with Akiva took place—was imagined as taking place—because Akiva had been arrested for participating in a revolt against the Romans and defying a ban against the study of Torah. He was sentenced to death. Stories have him reciting the Shema ("Hear, O Israel the Lord our God, the Lord is one") while Roman soldiers tore lumps of flesh from his body with iron combs.

2.

A DECADE AGO, I began to take a passionate interest in the Sabbath, the ancient weekly day of rest. I told myself that this was purely a matter of intellectual curiosity, but it wasn't. My feelings were murkier than that. I was ravenous for something, though I didn't know what. I tried to get my hands on everything having to do with the Sabbath. Tales of good Sabbaths and of bad Sabbaths. Angry screeds against the dour Sabbath ("Sunday comes, and brings with it a day of general gloom and austerity. The man who has been toiling hard all the week, has been looking towards the Sabbath, not as to a day of rest from labour, and healthy recreation, but as one of grievous tyranny and grinding oppression"—Charles Dickens) and fulsome praise for its blessings ("In the Universe of Shabbat, a person finds everything new, different, more elevated and exalted"—Dov Peretz Elkins).

Mine was not exactly a socially productive obsession. Saying that I'd been reading up on the Sabbath was a good way to cut a vigorous conversation short. Occasionally, some kind soul would agree to chat briefly about the great modern work on the subject, Rabbi Abraham Joshua Heschel's *The Sabbath*, a retelling of Hasidic legend that has become a popular primer for people taking their first steps back to Judaism. This is a beautiful book, but many of the others I could have talked about were not. The more I read about the Sabbath, though, the more I was struck by the power of the idea. It seemed to me that I could justify my interest in utilitarian terms. I could explain to my skeptical friends that a structured period of non-productivity could be very useful for an overscheduled society.

Soon after that, I came across another beautiful book. It was called *The Seven Day Circle*, by Eviatar Zerubavel, an American sociologist. Zerubavel grew up in Israel, a country where religious holidays are enforced with a strictness unusual in highly modernized societies. His immersion in the religious calendar had helped him to invent a whole new field, the sociology of time. Reading this book, I learned that the seven-day week was a by-product of the Jewish Sabbath. (The Israeli poet Chaim Nachman Bialik called the day "the most brilliant creation of the Hebrew spirit.") More important, I discovered that time has an architecture, and that that architecture has the power to affect us as deeply as the architecture of space does. Heschel wrote charming fables that revealed a world of legend inside the Sabbath. Zerubavel wrote dry social theory that made me grasp that even something as basic as the week has a history and an intoxicating power—the power to seem so natural that we don't realize how carefully constructed it has been. It made me eager to understand the shape of *my* week—where it came from, what it meant, what values it incarnated.

I remember the exact moment when I realized that I wanted to write a book on this unwieldy subject. I was closing a gate behind me. The gate led to the backyard of a lovely little Tudor-style cottage that belonged to the man who would become my husband. The inside of this house, with its sloped ceilings and plain furniture, put me in mind of an English country church. Heschel calls the Sabbath a cathedral in time. My future husband's house was a parsonage in the suburbs. We had just driven up from somewhere and I had been trying to explain to him what the Sabbath was, and why it mattered to Jews, and how it had once mattered terribly to Christians, too—particularly American Christians, and most particularly the American Puritans who founded this nation. They had such a deep hunger for the Sabbath—for the right *kind* of Sabbath—that they left England, whose Sabbaths they considered corrupt and lax, and sailed to America, in order to keep the kind of disciplined, godly Sabbaths they believed would transform their earthly existence into a New Jerusalem.

My future husband was a man with an impressive background in American history, but he didn't know about the role the Sabbath had played in it. He belonged to a synagogue, but he had never thought of the Sabbath as anything but an antiquated practice reserved for those with a masochistic taste for censorious laws. His face lit up, as it always does when he is given a fresh idea to mull over, and suddenly I saw what he saw: a largely forgotten aspect of the history of Western civilization and a non-academic way to explore an arcane but fascinating subject—that is to say, the social morality of time.

The social morality of time! I said. What a great phrase! No one thinks of time as a moral entity. We think of it as a mathematically neutral one. But what was the labor movement's fight for shorter days and workweeks about, if not the social morality of time? And how about the way we're always recalibrating our feelings for our friends, or our sense of how they feel about us, with the neurotic precision of a Larry David, based on how many minutes they've kept us waiting? If other people's use of our time isn't the object of infinitesimal ethical calculation, I don't know what is.

But that's not all the Sabbath is, I added. At this point he was opening the door to his house, which we knew, without ever having talked about it, I would soon be moving into. The Sabbath, I said, is not only an idea. It is also something you *keep.* With other people. You can't just extract lessons from it. Me, I want to keep it and teach my children to keep it. But at the same time, since I grew up watching a religious mother and a skeptical father play tug-of-war over our upbringing in a home in which the Sabbath was largely the occasion for unspoken recriminations about how we were being raised, I'm afraid that if I impose the Sabbath on my children they will resent me as much as I resented my parents. They will suss out signs of my ambivalence and use them as proof of my inconsistency and hypocrisy, as I did in my time. I like the *idea* of keeping the Sabbath, but at the thought of actually *doing* it, of passing an entire day following strange rules while refraining from customary recreations, I am knocked flat by a wave of anticipated boredom.

My soon-to-be fiancé looked baffled and a little worried: What was he getting himself into?

Religion is made up of rites and customs, I explained, or would have explained, had I thought of it at the time. These rites and customs get handed down like pieces of antique furniture, the names of their makers lost, their sentimental value forgotten along with the ancestors who treasured them. To dig up the meaning of this inheritance, to honor those ancestors and put myself in some sort of relation to them—that is what I want to do.

But to do that you have to give up so much! To do it right, at least as I construed "right" at the time. To submit to the rituals of the Sabbath and let them take you where they will, which is a place far beyond what Heschel called, with some irritation, "religious behaviorism" and "the sociological fallacy." By that, he meant the purely external understanding of religion as a set of behaviors and traditions worth preserving: religion construed as a social asset. To be transformed by a religious experience, rather than merely to appreciate it, to drop an anchor into the depths of the past and keep your life from drifting away, you have to be willing, I thought, to give yourself over to a different way of living, one that seems antiquated and foreign and extinguishing unless you're already immersed in it. You had to become that dreadful thing, *a religious person*.

I had always associated being religious with all sorts of unfortunate character traits. Being *really* religious, I mean. Because in my family we did not think of ourselves as religious. We kept the Sabbath by lighting candles and having dinner on Friday night. We kept kosher, sort of, at least in the house, by not mixing milk and meat and eating only kosher-slaughtered meat, though we didn't keep two sets of dishes, the way Orthodox Jews do, and all of us except my mother ate whatever we liked in restaurants or at other people's houses, although she sometimes muttered things about having failed as a parent when we ordered pork or shrimp. We did what our parents did and they did what their parents did, largely in defiance of *their* parents, with their old-world styles of observance. Apart from my mother, there was no one around to care whether it was done in the prescribed manner—and even she didn't care enough to stop us from breaking the rules.

Religiosity, to us, was obsessive-compulsive, masochistic, intellectually narrow, irrational, tribalistic, antimodern. Living the religious life, especially the Jewish religious life, means making a commitment to live by rules that are neither logical nor natural. Why should we only eat animals that chew their cud and have cloven hooves? Why are we forbidden to wear clothes that mix wool and flax? You have to take these rules on faith, and derive their legitimacy from tradition. To become religious is to brave a leap into the absurd. Kierkegaard understood that to be a terrible leap. You have to bow to that which is commanded. You have to give up your ability to control your world. It's a form of self-sacrifice. Kierkegaard compares it to Abraham's sacrifice of Isaac.

Kierkegaard couldn't make the leap. He could describe the movements of faith, he said, but he couldn't perform them. They were, he said, like hanging by the waist from a belt attached to the ceiling and making the gestures people make when they're swimming. He could tell us what the gestures of faith were, but if he were thrown into the waters of belief he would not be able to swim the way one who had faith would swim—whatever way that might be. (Kierkegaard isn't very good at describing it.) But he did admire the faithful.

The problem was—Kierkegaard went on—that he had never met a man of true faith. To uncover the meaning of the religious experience, therefore, he has to make such a man up. He imagines he meets a man whom he recognizes instantly as "a knight of faith." To his amazement, this man betrays absolutely no connection to a higher order of things. His façade has no "crack from which the infinite peeped out." He looks like a member of the petite bourgeoisie. He looks, in fact, like a tax collector. And one way in which he expresses his petite bourgeoisie-ness is by keeping the Sabbath: "He takes a holiday on Sundays. He goes to church." He sings the psalms lustily, but offers up no other sign of exceptionality. In the afternoon he takes a walk in the woods, delighting in everything he sees. On the way home, he thinks about his wife and the "special warm little dish" she will have prepared for him. He engages in various other small pleasures and has minor social interactions, including an exchange that might drum up some real-estate business. In the evening, he smokes his pipe: "To see him you would swear it was the cheesemonger opposite vegetating in the dusk." And yet, Kierkegaard continued, "and yet—yes, it could drive me to fury, out of envy if for no other reason—and yet this man has made and is at every moment making the movement of infinity."

Kierkegaard did not home in on his stolid burgher's Sabbath by accident. There is no better point of entry to the religious experience than the Sabbath, for all its apparent ordinariness. *Because* of its ordinariness. The extraordinariness of the Sabbath lies in its being commonplace. We who look at religion from the outside think of transcendence as something that occurs at special moments, in concentrated bursts of illumination, but people raised in homes where religious ritual occurs over breakfast and at dinner and in school and throughout weekends know that revelation commingles promiscuously with routine. If ritual is art, then it is stretched over the frame of habit.

This is particularly true of the Judaism reinvented by the rabbinic sages, whose masterwork, the Talmud, an enormous anthology of all their legal and theological debates, transformed a temple-based religion suited to a pastoral and agricultural people into a ritual-based religion suited to an urban and far-flung one. In their Judaism, just about every activity in the day has its own blessing, and many of them follow in a carefully choreographed sequence. There are blessings for waking up, for washing the hands, for eating bread or water, for going to the bathroom. In a study of the rabbinic mind, the philosopher Max Kadushin called holiness a "normal mysticism." It isn't "necessarily associated with the unusual and the awesome," he wrote. "On the contrary, it may be centered on personal conduct and be associated with the ordinary and familiar." The rabbis demystified holiness; they democratized it, making it less a function of spiritual genius than of personal self-discipline.

If you view the stuff of everyday life as the raw material of Judaism, and its rules as a framing device, then you will grasp something essential about the Sabbath: It is meant to turn the ordinary into the singular. A weekly house scrubbing, when done on Friday, becomes a way of making one's home ready for God. A dinner party for family and neighbors attains the status of a royal banquet, welcoming home the Sabbath queen. To the mundane satisfaction that comes from cultivating good habits—cleanliness, organization, family togetherness—

is added the sublime sense of rightness that comes from following God's commandments.

Keeping the Sabbath, I felt, would be good for me. It would force me to grow up and take my place among the generations. It would charge my domestic middle-aged life with drama and significance, whereas now it felt drained and resigned. But in order for this to happen I would have to stop feeling so ambivalent about the day.

3.

BUT WAS IT JUST ME who was uncomfortable with the Sabbath? Or is it intrinsically discomfiting in some way?

Whenever I ask myself this question, I come back to Kierkegaard's tax collector. It's funny how he pops up just as Kierkegaard is worrying about the impossibility of attaining the faith of Abraham, a figure of indescribable heroism and fathomless trust, who was asked to destroy all that was good, all that he had waited for and loved, and yet somehow never doubted his God. That the only character Kierkegaard can conjure up for his latter-day "knight of faith" is a "philistine" (as the philosopher calls him) suggests that the man is not so much a beau ideal as a product of Kierkegaard's irrepressible irony (even though Kierkegaard regarded irony as an attribute of lower natures). The tax collector's "movement of infinity" turns out to be a movement of finite this-worldiness and external ceremonial. The tax collector is supposed to embody Abraham—he's the modern Abraham—but turns out to be his opposite.

And then two more thoughts occur to me. First, when Kierkegaard chose Abraham to exemplify the paradox of faith he was making use of a very old Christian interpretation of the patriarch, according to which Abraham incarnated the higher spirituality that the Jews lost when they bound themselves to the Torah, with its physical fetishes and weird commandments. Abraham proved that faith was greater than law, for he left his home and his religion and nearly sacrificed his son Isaac, all without the crutch of ritual. Abraham prefigured Christ, who died so that those who came after him could live by faith, not by law. Abraham, by this reading, was the father of the Christians, not of the Jews, who had repudiated him.

And, second, I am struck by the fact that Kierkegaard made his "knight of faith" a tax collector. To compare the accursed tax collector to the blessed Abraham is—given the long association of Jews with the handling of money, not to mention tax collection—to make *him* the Jew, rather than Abraham, the father of Christians. It is to imbue his carnal Sabbath with the gross corporality that befouls the body of the stereotypical Jew. The incredulity in Kierkegaard's voice is that this improbably, laughably *Jewy* character should be the "knight of faith."

You can always count on Franz Kafka to get the joke, and to push it one step further. In a letter to his best friend, Max Brod, Kafka complained of *Fear and Trembling*—which he loved—that Kierkegaard is blind to Abraham "the ordinary man," the Abraham who *did* have elements of the philistine in him. Kierkegaard, instead, gives us "this monstrous Abraham in the clouds." Kafka had another Abraham to propose, a comical Abraham, who is, in fact, exactly as picayune and rule-bound as the "knight of faith," except that he's also neurotic, overeager, Woody Allenesque. He just can't stop getting ready for the big day, his sacrifice of Isaac. This is an Abraham, Kafka wrote elsewhere, who "would be ready to fulfill the demand of the sacrifice immediately, with the promptness of a waiter, but who could not bring off the sacrifice, because he can't get away from the house, he is indispensable, the household needs him, there is always something more to put in order, the house is not ready." This Abraham is like a Jew obsessively getting ready for the Sabbath, a Jew bogged down in the physical details of spiritual preparation.

Everyone knows that Christians, early and late, have had mixed feelings about Jews. It is less well known that they have had mixed feelings about the Sabbath. More than mixed feelings, they had questions: Would Christ have wanted them to keep it? If so, how strictly? Did they *really* have to worry about the innumerable rules? Or was the Sabbath just too *Jewish,* a discardable artifact of Jewish "chosenness," antithetical to the spirit of the new universal religion? There are many complex explanations for their uncertainty, but there is also a simple explanation. The simple one takes us back to the interpreters and followers of the apostle Paul, who said that Christ had superseded the "ceremonial," or purely physical, external aspects of the Law, making it permissible for Christians to keep only its "moral" or spiritual components. (What Paul himself said is harder to suss out.) The one Old Testament ceremony that resisted supersession, however, was the Sabbath. For even though in the Gospels Christ objected to its overpunctilious observance—"The Sabbath was made for man, and not man for the Sabbath," he told the Pharisees who scowled at his disciples' Sabbath violations—he appears, on the whole, to have kept it. Moreover, the Sabbath was the only ritual law among the Ten Commandments, which Christians have held to be universal or natural laws—that is, a kind of innate morality implanted by God in the human soul. But the Old Testament called the Sabbath a sign of the covenant between God and the Jews. It was particular to them, not to mention peculiar, and not easily alchemized into something universal. And yet there it was, number four on the list.

At this point I'd better step back and try to define the Sabbath. As I'm using the term, it's the day in the week on which Jews and Christians (at least those who accept the Sabbath) are commanded not to work. It is the execution of a set of ritual proscriptions and prescriptions, the proscriptions largely having to do with work and the prescriptions largely having to do with making the day worshipful and festive. It is derived from the Fourth Commandment: "Remember the sabbath day, to keep it holy. Six days shalt thou labour, and do all thy work: But the seventh day is the sabbath of the Lord thy God: in it thou shalt not do any work, thou, nor thy son, nor thy daughter, thy manservant, nor thy maidservant, nor thy cattle, nor thy stranger that is within thy gates."

By this definition, I should add, the holy day called Al-Jumuah, which Muslims celebrate on Friday, cannot be considered a Sabbath, though it is sometimes said to be the Muslim Sabbath. The scholarly footnotes in my Koran insist firmly on this point. Al-Jumuah is not a day of non-work, nor is it necessarily a time for socializing inside or outside the mosque. It is an hour or so of prayer, accompanied by a weekly sermon. Shortly before noon, Muslim store owners shutter their stores and workers leave their offices and places of employment for the service—in New York City, taxicabs line the streets outside mosques—but on the whole they return to work a few hours later. One Muslim teaching reads: "When the time for Jumu'ah prayer comes, close your business and answer the summons loyally and earnestly, meet earnestly, pray, consult, and learn by social contact: when the meeting is over, scatter and go about your business."

I should also add that the image we hold in our heads of the Jewish Sabbath isn't wholly based on the Fourth Commandment, either. The Sabbath of candlelighting and dinners and not driving and not turning lights on and off was shaped more by rabbinic law than by the Torah. This Sabbath may have been practiced in Christ's time, but it was codified in the Talmud in the centuries following his crucifixion. This law identifies thirty-nine main categories of work that may not be done from the moment the Sabbath begins until it ends, unless the life of an individual or the welfare of a community is at stake. There are countless subcategories of the categories, and innumerable permutations of those. *Shabbat,* the Talmudic tractate, or book about the Sabbath, is the longest of all the tractates in the Talmud, and there's another tractate devoted entirely to the law of Sabbath boundaries, called *Eruvin.* "There are one hundred and fifty-seven two-sided pages in tractate Sabbath, and one hundred and five in Eruvin," the Israeli poet Bialik complained, notwithstanding his admiration for the Sabbath. "For the most part they consist of discussions and decisions on the minutiae of the thirty-nine kinds of work and their branches. . . . What weariness of flesh! What waste of good wits on every trifling point!"

How *can* Jews bear to obey all these laws? Well, why does any society adhere to its customs? These rituals make sense to Jews because being members of their community means being committed to making sense of them. The Law—Torah—is the language Jews use to speak to one another. It is their way of discussing the mandated acts, inherited traditions, and interpersonal obligations that make up any discernibly discrete cultural group. It is a Jew's commitment to the ongoing process of Law, of studying and interpreting and reinterpret-ing—and following—the laws, that brings out the aspect of the Law that is world-creating, rather than soul-stifling. Besides, the Law is said to make God's will manifest, and following it is not thought to be a burden (though it may be experienced as such) but the chance to make God's transcendental goodness a reality on earth.

By the time the rabbis began writing their books on the Jewish Sabbath, however, Christians had on the whole (though not entirely) cut themselves off from Jewish communities. Many Christians had never had any contact with Jews to begin with. The Jewish Sabbath had stopped making sense to them, and had stopped being made sense of by them. Paul had already told Gentile converts that Moses' Law was a dead weight on them, a yoke to be cast off. The theologi-cal principle of supersession expressed a sociological fact. The Chris-tians had moved on. Yet they still lugged the Sabbath around with them.

I first grasped what it must have felt like to have to carry the Sab-bath around like a suitcase full of stuff you don't need anymore but are unable to drop into a dumpster while I was having a small fit of petu-lance about having to get up from my desk and go to see my psycho-analyst. Now, like, say, rabbinic Judaism during the time of medieval Christendom, psychoanalysis is considered an anachronism. Who has the time or the money to undergo analysis anymore? Who believes in its efficacy? Well, I do, or at least I have a superstitious inability to stop seeing my analyst. But when I do so I often find myself mumbling grumpily to myself about her and all her rules. As I boarded my train, glancing anxiously at my watch, it occurred me that the psychoana-lytic session, with its rules and rhythm and punctuality, is a modern Sabbath.

The psychoanalytic session, like the Sabbath, takes you out of mundane time and forces you into what might be called sacred time—the timeless time of the unconscious, with its yawning infantile unboundedness, its shattered sequentiality. It may not be pleasant, it may not be convenient, you may not want to go, but you do. On time. And the fixed time limits also keep you from losing yourself in that disorienting, disorganizing flux. When your fifty minutes are up, you return to the mercilessness of the regular week. But your fifty minutes will come around again, just as mercilessly, and you must present yourself on time or give an account of yourself.

The Sabbath is an organizing principle. It is a socially reinforced temporal structure. Either you want to be organized in this way or you don't, or, if you're like me, you do and you don't. But if you're like me you can't quite forget what it feels like to have a Sabbath. You can tell when it's missing, even if you don't necessarily miss it.

4.

AMERICANS, ONCE THE MOST Sabbatarian people on earth, are now the most ambivalent on the subject. On the one hand, we miss the Sabbath. When we pine for escape from the rat race; when we check into spas, yoga centers, encounter weekends, spiritual retreats; when we fret about the disappearance of a more old-fashioned time, with its former, generally agreed-upon rhythms of labor and repose; when we deplore the increase in time devoted to consumption; when we complain about the commercialization of leisure, which turns fun into work and requires military-scale budgeting and logistics and interactions with service personnel—whenever we worry about these things, we are remembering the Sabbath, its power to protect us from the clamor of our own desires. But when, say, we return from a trip to some less developed country and feel a sense of relief that our twenty-four-hour economy allows us to work, shop, dine, and be entertained when *we* want to, not according to some imposed schedule, at that point, too, we are remembering the Sabbath. We are remembering how claustrophobic its rigid temporal boundaries used to make us feel.

This book is about my ambivalence toward the Sabbath, which I diagnose as partly the secular American's ambivalence toward the Sabbath and partly an ambivalence peculiarly my own. It is my theory that these ambivalences can be traced in some way to the Christian ambivalence toward the Sabbath, which can be traced in some way to a deeper ambivalence toward the idea of living a life in thrall to law and tradition, which can be traced in some way to an even deeper ambivalence toward ritual, which can be traced in some way to the most profound possible qualms about holiness, an uncanny, spectral quality that forces itself upon us from its perch in the past. All these *in some ways* should tip you off that this book is more associative than analytical and more anecdotal than historical (though there is analysis and history in it).

This book is also, to use an execrable expression, a journey—not a conversion narrative, in which the journey begins *here* and ends *there,* but an inconclusive account of a life led in the shadow of the Sabbath, and of the texts and ideas I've read in an effort to make sense of its strange possession. This is not a work of journalism, either. I have spent many Sabbaths with many people—Orthodox Jews, Seventh-Day Adventists—and I have always felt what Kierkegaard felt, which is that watching from the outside raises more questions than it answers. The great writer Alice Munro puts it even better than Kierkegaard does: "Only from the inside of the faith is it possible to get any idea of the prize as well as the struggle, the addictive pursuit of pure righteousness, the intoxication of a flash of God's favor."

So I've looked inside my Sabbath, compromised as it is, for some sense of the prize and the struggle, and I've tried to steal glimpses into the Sabbaths of history—the ones that happened to interest me, rather than the ones that are objectively considered to be the most important. Sometimes, to get a better look, I've stuck a sort of periscope out the window, using sociology or anthropology or even economics to give myself a longer view and ask and try to answer questions deeper than those I would have dared to pose in face-to-face interviews. I've organized this book around some of the themes that swam into view. I hope I've done this without succumbing to the fantasy that the use of these elevated terminologies lends my musings the patina of truth. This is, in the end, a work of apologetics, even though I'm still trying to get over the feeling that I have to apologize for that fact.

THE SABBATH WORLD

PART ONE

Time Sickness

1.

IN THE POETRY OF THE PRAYER BOOK, THE SABBATH IS A BRIDE GREETED by an impatient bridal party with an almost anguished relief. In the more prosaic dominion of my house, the Sabbath sees herself in and sits down to wait. As the woman of the house, and, more to the point, the only person in my family whose heart pounds anxiously at the approach of a religious obligation, it's up to me to acknowledge her presence by lighting the candles eighteen minutes before sunset, when they should be lit. During the winter, however, I don't light the candles on time. I ignore the clock at the bottom of my computer screen and when I don't see the numbers turn to, say, 4:10, I don't look out the window, where the shadows of our trees are beginning to black out the backyard.

I know without looking, though, that the room where the candles would be burning is having its last golden moment of the day, the sun having sunk low enough to gild the walls. The sun sets shortly thereafter and plunges the world inside my time zone into what Jewish tradition regards as a kind of temporal no-man's-land. It's neither the end of the sixth day nor the beginning of the seventh (the Jewish day beginning and ending at nightfall). It's twilight. The rabbis, who mixed their prescriptions and proscriptions with legend, defined twilight as "from sunset as long as the face of the east has a reddish glow." They also called the twilight before the Sabbath a witching hour. The story is told that on the very first Sabbath twilight God created ten magical objects that he would later use to make miracles: the rainbow that came after the flood to assure mankind that God wouldn't destroy the world again; the staff with which Moses wrought the ten plagues; the mouth of the earth that opened up to swallow an Israelite who tried to launch a coup against Moses; and so on.

By the time I'm ready to enter the kitchen and start my Sabbath, the moment for miracles will have passed. So will my chance to cheat time. The rabbis were inflexible about punctuality. The Romans having leveled the Temple more than a century before the rabbis became the Jews' highest religious authorities, the sages inherited an inoperative religion of space, and set about turning it into a religion of time. It's no accident that in the very first passage of the Talmud, they try to determine the exact instant in the evening after which a Jew may say the Shema, the most important prayer in Judaism. To the rabbis, time is irreversible. Generally speaking, either you do things at the appointed time or you don't do them at all.

Such is the magic of the twilight before the Sabbath, though, that for that moment the march of time pauses in mid-step. The Jew may no longer light candles, but he or she may complete a few last preparations. Of course, the rabbis disagreed about how long this reprieve should last. Is it still twilight if the lower half of the horizon is dark but the upper half is still red? Maybe a more precise measure is the time it takes for a man to walk half a *mil* (three-quarters of a mile). Finally, one nervous adjudicator declared that twilight is "as the twinkling of an eye" and impossible to define, so you should never do even what is permitted at twilight lest the Sabbath has already come and you violate it accidentally.

Nonetheless, the twilight before the Sabbath is an exception to the time-bound nature of most Jewish obligations, and, like most exceptions, it underscores the rule. Jewish law is like musical notation; it gives meaning to the stuff of life by regulating it in time. The Sabbath is its most sacred interval. That I can't subsume my schedule to its sterner rhythms testifies, I feel, to a flaw in my character. But it also says something about how hard it is for a twenty-first-century American to accept being governed by a calendar so firmly bolted down to the ground that she doesn't get to move it around, adjust it by an hour here, an hour there. A rabbi who no longer works at the synagogue in the small suburban town where I no longer live once horrified its congregants by insisting that if they couldn't get home to light the candles on time they shouldn't light them at all. This struck everyone as harsh, not to mention impolitic, since a large part of the modern rabbi's job is to woo apostates back into the fold.

The old-time Sabbath does not fit comfortably into our lives. It scowls at our dewy dreams of total relaxation and freedom from obligation. The goal of the Sabbath may be rest, but it isn't personal liberty or unfettered leisure. The Sabbath seems designed to make life as inconvenient as possible. Our schedules are not the only thing the Sabbath would disrupt if it could. It would also rip a hole in all the shimmering webs that give modern life its pleasing aura of weightlessness—the networks that zap digitized voices and money and data from server to iPhone to GPS. In a world of brightness and portability and instantaneous intimacy, the Sabbath foists on the consciousness the blackness of night, the heaviness of objects, the miles that keep us apart. The Sabbath prefers natural to artificial light. If we want to travel, it would make us walk, though not too far. If we long for social interaction, it would have us meet our fellow man and woman face-to-face. If we wish to bend the world to our will, it would insist that we forgo the vast majority of the devices that extend our reach and multiply our efficacy. We would be deprived of money and, to a certain degree, of the labor of others. We would be allowed to use our hands and a few utensils, and then only for a limited repertoire of activities. There is something gorgeously naïve about the Sabbath. To forbid people their tools and machines and commercial transactions, to reduce their social contacts to those who live no more than a village's distance away—it seems a child's idea, really, of life before civilization. Human existence, by the time it became human, was never that concrete.

According to sociologists, modern life is complex. Indeed, to them, the word *modern* implies complexity. Our lives get their feeling of disjointedness from the fact that our social networks—family, profession, church, neighborhood—don't fit neatly inside one another like Chinese boxes, as, supposedly, they did in premodern times. That means we often play several mutually conflicting roles, navigate among thousands of cross-cultural expectations, employ hundreds of thousands of systems of communication, from linguistic and gestural and sartorial to electronic and financial, in the course of a single day. On the other hand, I can't imagine that life in the ancient world was much simpler. True, biblical man and woman had a more fixed place in the world. Their social circles were less segmented and contrapuntal. But men and women still had to feed and clothe and shelter themselves and their children. They had to get along with relatives and neighbors and authority figures; they had to contend with strangers and foreign aggressors. They had to achieve competence in all the social strategies required to secure status and resources and pass those on to their children. They lived in the world, not in the Garden of Eden.

The rabbis say that the Sabbath is a taste of the world to come. Me, I think it's an aftertaste of infancy. It's a fantasy of perfect wholeness. If adult life is divided, the Sabbath is when we become one—with our family, with our community, with God. The Kabbalists say that on the Sabbath each of us is granted an additional soul, a *neshama yeterah*. I imagine that oversoul as a big, fleecy blanket.

2.

IT WAS, I THINK, that primal warmth, what Freud called religion's oceanic feeling, that my mother was trying to summon up when she made Shabbat for us children. She wanted us to have the honey-tinged Friday-night experience described in our children's books. But the event she choreographed could not have been less heartwarming, because my mother, when we arrived in Puerto Rico, went away— not physically, but her unhappiness made our apartment feel evacuated. She hated our beach condo and kept it clean with a mechanical efficiency, her thin lips pursed, her once fluffy curls limp with the wet salt air. She answered all questions with a bitter laugh. Her tone with salesmen and checkout clerks quivered with barely contained rage.

My father fled every morning to the industrial-laundry facility he was building in the suburbs; when he returned in the evening, he avoided her gaze and complained about the inefficiency of his Puerto Rican employees.

My mother had once dreamed of making aliyah—moving to Israel—and San Juan, to her, was about as far from Jerusalem as you could get. Friday night was the culmination of a week of hating her life. She would round up her reluctant husband and children, light her candles, and say the blessing over the wine and challah. When she said the kiddush, which in those days was strictly a man's job, my father would signal his boredom by fiddling with the silverware. As she served dinner, she would force her voice to grow mellow, but it would soon grow tight and bitter. She launched us into grace after the meal with an officious air that accused us of having abandoned her.

The Sabbath was the opposite of a refuge in time. And yet refuge was what I craved most. My earliest memory of Puerto Rico involves light. In Detroit, sunlight had had a gentle, autumnal tinge. I can see the pavement now as if from my stroller, edged in a faded Kodak red the color of fallen leaves. In San Juan, the sidewalks were relentlessly white. To walk to school, I crossed a street just short of where it ended on a beach, the waves breaking in a gleaming spray. Then I cut through a parking lot between two buildings and followed Ashford Avenue, the main thoroughfare, as it curved along the shore, lined by one boxy albino condominium building after another. The school, a pale-green cinder-block construction, glowed helplessly in the sun.

Some crucial sense of shelter had vanished from my life. The year we arrived, my parents sent me to kindergarten at an American school in the suburbs. The first time I took the bus, the bus driver walked back to my seat and asked me my name so that he could look up my address on his roster. I couldn't tell him. I didn't remember my first name, and I didn't remember my last name. Nor could I remember what part of town I lived in. I sat in the front row, mute with embarrassment, as he deposited every other child at his or her destination. Then we drove all the way back to school to find someone who could call my parents to come and get me. I nearly peed on the leatherette seat.

The Talmud asks, What if a person is traveling in the desert and forgets which day is Shabbat and there's no one around to tell him? The answer takes the form of a dispute, as do all answers in the Talmud. One rabbi says the man should count six days from the day he first realizes he doesn't know what day it is, then keep the seventh as the Sabbath. Another rabbi says no, he should keep the Sabbath on the very next day, then count six more before he keeps it again. Missing from this bizarrely numerical discussion is any acknowledgment of the desperation of someone in that situation. How lost do you have to be to forget which day it is?

When I first read this passage, I immediately thought of the aviator in Antoine de Saint-Exupéry's *The Little Prince,* a beloved book of my childhood. Can the ancient traveler be as isolated as a man who has crashed in the middle of the Sahara, "a thousand miles from any inhabited territory," not to mention from food and water, a man who may or may not be hallucinating when he encounters a little boy in a swallow-tailed coat who has himself fallen from the too-bright sky?

The rabbis, I like to believe, were sufficiently acquainted with exile that they could imagine feeling as cut off as the aviator, and in their wisdom they understood that all you have left under those conditions is fantasy. For what they ask you to do, when you have lost the world, is to make one up. Another rabbi asks, How are we to understand the rabbi who says count six then keep one? He wants us to count as God counted when he was creating the world. And how are we to understand the second rabbi, the one who says to keep the Sabbath then count six more days? We are to count the way Adam counted. He was created on the sixth day and God rested on the seventh, so the first thing Adam did was rest.

The question underlying the dispute, I think, is this: When time has disappeared and space is a comfortless ripple of white sand, should you imagine yourself inside the skin of the first man or inside the mind of God? The Talmud gives an answer to this question. It is, the mind of God. To save yourself, you re-create the world.

3.
———

THE FIRST URGES to keep the Sabbath came over me sometime after college. I was unable to settle on anything to do on Friday nights and would spend Saturdays alone, away from my busy, brunching friends. It took me years to grasp that there was a link between my Friday nights present and past. Trying to keep the Sabbath, I thought, would give me something to do when melancholy set in. It would serve as a therapeutic subordination of the self. But I never really got around to subordinating myself, at least not to the level of Orthodoxy I considered (without ever having quite admitted this fact to myself) the authentic mode of self-subordination. So now, when I come into the house and find my children freshly bathed but not dressed, dinner uncooked, and the table unset, I feel light-headed with self-disgust.

If only I'd been raised in a fully traditional home, instead of my half-godless one! If only I had been trained to follow rules, rather than having been spoiled by the modern disrespect for them! On the other hand, who has time for all these rules? Like anyone else trying to get ahead, before I had children I logged late hours and weekends in the office, then complained proudly to my friends. When my children were little, I rushed irritably through every diaper change, every walk, every meal. There seemed no other way to retain economic independence, professional viability, a feeling of competence, the faith that I would continue to exist once I stepped outside the house. Observing the Sabbath as it was supposed to be observed seemed strictly aspirational.

In short, for me, the Sabbath is not, and never has been, a day of rest. It is a torturous dangle between two orders of, well, time, though I'm not sure that word captures the degree of incompatibility I have in mind. The Sabbath is the place where the modern and mundane open up to yield glimpses of something else—something half monk-ish and half Romantic and wholly imaginary. But, just at the moment that I am about to enter this world, I hear my father's voice. It tells me that I am freer than any Jew who came before me. I'm not restricted to Jewish schools and workplaces. I don't have to obey oppressive Jewish rules. Why twist freedom into a curse?

4.

IN 1919, shortly after the end of World War I, a Hungarian neurolo-gist named Sándor Ferenczi, a disciple and close friend of Sigmund Freud's, identified a new disorder, the "Sunday neurosis," which he defined as "mostly *headaches* or *stomach disturbances* that were wont to appear on this day without any particular cause, and often utterly spoilt the young people's one free day of the week." After ruling out possible physical causes, such as overeating and oversleeping, Ferenczi decided that his patients were having a problem with the day itself.

Ferenczi's essay is now considered to be the first description of workaholism, but Ferenczi thought that it reflected the relationship between mental illness and time. He was diagnosing a time sickness. "We know from psychiatry," he wrote, "of illnesses that display a marked periodicity. . . . But as far as I am aware no one has yet de-scribed neuroses the oscillation of whose symptoms were dependent on the particular day of the week."

In this, Ferenczi predicted the future. Nearly a century later, spe-cialists in a new field, chronobiology, study the internal clocks of liv-ing things, which are driven by an intricate dance of outside and inside factors—by light and darkness interacting with hormones. Cortisol, the so-called stress hormone, floods our bodies in the morn-ing, waking us up, and drains out of them at night, allowing us to relax. An unhappy evening can disrupt the rhythm of cortisol release, making it hard for us to sleep, which can, in turn, make us depressed or exacerbate our already fragile grip on reality. Melatonin is the hormone that ensures a normal sleep-wake cycle. Usually we make melatonin at night. But if night disappears as a result of indoor lighting our glands won't know when it's time to start working, and we'll have more sleep problems.

Most of these biological rhythms have roughly a twenty-four-hour cycle, though some, like menstruation, have a monthly cycle, and some correspond to the seasons. There are also what are known as circaseptan, or about-weekly, rhythms, although so far more of these have been spotted in small marine creatures than in people. Medical studies have uncovered seven-day patterns in blood pressure and migraines, though it is unclear whether these are rooted in social experience or genomes—one study found that people have fewer migraines on Sunday than on any other day of the week. Sociologists and psychiatrists have spotted many seven-day behavioral patterns— suicides famously skyrocket on Mondays; dreams tend to incorporate images a week old or less—but these patterns mirror social realities, not the activity of our cells. Depressives kill themselves on Mondays because the workday's seemingly unmanageable routines drown them in despair. We file short-term memories in seven-day chunks because that's how we're used to thinking.

Chronobiology may be on the verge of proving that the week exists in nature, but for the moment the seven-day cycle remains a social unit of time—in a way, the very first. The week was the first temporal division not tethered to the sun or the moon. It was the first calendrical algorithm, rolling forward into the future according to its own logic and with no regard for the rotations of the astral bodies. "So long as man marked his life only by the cycles of nature," the historian Daniel Boorstin wrote, "he remained a prisoner of nature. If he was to go his own way and fill his world with human novelties, he would have to make his own measures of time."

If the week is a socially constructed measure of time, then when people get sick every Sunday their illness is probably not a biological

disorder. It's a reaction to Sunday itself. But what about the day pro-
vokes this reaction? "Sunday is the holiday of present-day civilized
humanity," Ferenczi explained. What made Sunday civilized, he declared, was that it was bacchanalian. To illustrate this paradox, Ferenczi imagined a Sunday that a person might spend with friends and
family. (You have to remember how literary and whimsical psychoanalysts allowed themselves to be in those days.) His illustrative fantasy
is very fin de siècle, very late Austro-Hungarian empire. It involves a
picnic in the mountains, where "everything is permissible." Adults
disport themselves like children. The children get wild and spiral out
of control. But not every adult will enjoy his "holiday wantonness."
Hilarity, in the Sunday neurotic, prompts self-loathing, not release. He
clamps down on himself, and his urges spill out as symptoms. During
the other days of the week, a busy schedule and strict codes of behavior keep dark feelings in check. On Sunday, when time loses its structure and conventions relax, they emerge.

Aha! I thought. So the goyim twist their freedom into a curse,
too! But then I read on, and noticed something strange. Aside from
this one made-up Sunday, Ferenczi bases his diagnosis entirely on a
single example set not on Sunday but on Friday night: a Jewish patient who remembered that, as a little boy, he vomited every Sabbath
eve. His family blamed the fish they usually had for dinner, but Ferenczi had another theory. "It is known that for religious Jews on Friday night, it is not just eating fish that is obligatory; so is marital love,"
he wrote. He was alluding to a rabbinic recommendation that couples
have sex on the Sabbath. What really disturbed his patient, Ferenczi
said, was that as a boy he had overheard his parents acting on that sug-
gestion and made himself sick to quash the thought that his beloved
mother could do *that* with his father.

When I first read Ferenczi's Oedipal explanation, it struck me as
crude, even ludicrous. How could the depth and complexity of the
boy's Friday-night experience be reduced to a groan overheard by
chance? But, given how prescient Ferenczi is in other respects, I decided to give him the benefit of the doubt. I also decided to look into
how he came to write that essay.

Most of what is known about Ferenczi comes from two decades' worth of letters to and from Freud. From them we learn that although Ferenczi, like Freud, was the kind of assimilated Jew whose idea of Sabbath rest meant Sunday sociability, he would have been perfectly well aware of the difference between Saturday and Sunday. Ferenczi grew up in a Jewish community in Miskolcz, a town in Hungary, where his mother probably lit Sabbath candles on Friday night. Both of Ferenczi's parents came from Poland, a country whose pious Jews made Hungary's less strict Jewish community look practically Christian. His mother was the president of a local organization of Jewish women and probably observant. His father, an ardent Hungarian nationalist and pamphleteer who changed his name from Fraenkel, probably wasn't.

By the time Ferenczi got to Budapest, at the turn of the twentieth century, it had grown into a gleaming metropolis on whose elegant boulevards promenaded writers, artists, and intellectuals, whose ranks soon included Ferenczi himself. They considered their city a Central European Paris where Sundays were for wrapping your arm around a lover's waist and strolling through a park; drinking and listening to bands in one of Budapest's big, gilded cafés; gathering with your family for a rich, desultory Sunday dinner; fleeing the heat with a trip to the nearby mountains. It was not a day of solemn prayer. Ferenczi saw patients on Saturdays. On Sundays, he usually took the train to Vienna to talk things over with Freud. He would not have wanted his diagnosis to reek of a parochial Jewishness. He wanted it to express the human condition. So maybe when he turned this Saturday neurosis into a Sunday one, he was, like the early Christian thinkers, universalizing. This is not to say that Ferenczi was anti-Jewish. On the contrary, he was a Jewish chauvinist, often bragging about the accomplishments of fellow members of the tribe. But he recoiled from everything having to do with Jewish ritual. So did Freud.

It's hard to remember now, but a century ago psychoanalysts like Freud and Ferenczi were going to rid the world of superstition and replace it with a fearless science of the self. They were going to forge the personality the sociologist Philip Rieff would later call "psychological man," the self-scrutinizing figure whose quest for individual self-improvement banished the more community-minded soul of previous eras. Psychological men and women had liberated their "I"'s. They had no time for the "we" cultivated by believers. Religion was a sickness, and Freud had come to cure it.

When Ferenczi blurred Saturday into Sunday, he may also have been worrying about anti-Semitism, which he and Freud feared would damn their new science to oblivion. In November 1917, less than six months before he sent Freud a finished draft of "Sunday Neurotics," Ferenczi dropped him a note announcing with relief that he was finally starting to see non-Jewish patients. He and Freud would both have interpreted this as a sign that psychoanalysis was becoming respectable in Hungary. On the other hand, this wouldn't have left Ferenczi time to psychoanalyze many Christians before sending his article to Freud. So where did he get his material? From Jewish patients, of course, and, I can't help suspecting, from himself. Like all the early analysts, Ferenczi was given to autobiographical reflection, and considered himself as good a subject of clinical study as anyone else.

Actually, I don't think it matters much whether he was talking about himself or someone else. Ferenczi's patients, it turns out, were a lot like him. They belonged to the first generation of Hungarian Jews to be admitted to Hungarian schools and universities—luckily for them, at a moment when these institutions happened to be unusually good—and granted free access to the professions. Historians refer to them as Hungary's golden generation. Some of them transcended the confines of Hungarian (one of the world's most difficult languages, and little read outside the country) and achieved world renown; among them were the composer Béla Bartók, the playwright Ferenc Molnár, the journalists Theodor Herzl and Arthur Koestler, the sociologist Karl Mannheim, the literary critic and philosopher Georg Lukács, and Ferenczi himself. The parents and grandparents of this generation had made their way to Budapest from poorer and more pious regions. They had kept their accents and many of their customs, even when they joined reformist synagogues that made rituals optional. (Throughout the nineteenth century, Hungary had a large, dynamic reform movement, called Neolog Judaism, that had much in common with the Reform Judaism prevalent in America at the same time.)

The poets, painters, and thinkers among them, critical of capitalism and the damage wrought on the countryside by industrialization, wrote and painted nostalgic visions of the villages of their (or their parents') childhood, but they had no desire to follow the religion practiced in them. They disliked the authoritarianism of faith; they cherished the newfound freedom of reason. The sight of black-hatted Eastern Jews, or *Ostjuden,* made these children particularly nervous. "My father, who otherwise never went to temple and certainly never prayed, once a year took me to some secret ceremony," reads one anxious passage in the memoir of the poet Béla Balázs, Ferenczi's contemporary. Balázs was talking about Yom Kippur, the holiest day in the Jewish calendar. "There were only men there whom I did not know and with whom my parents did not socialize. With white sheets on their shoulders, they wailed and beat their breasts. But what was really frightening for me was that my father too donned such a white sheet, which was edged with black stripes, and dressed like them, he joined and entered this alien and secret alliance."

So maybe it's not enough to say that Ferenczi's patient associated fish with his parents having sex or that he had an existential dread of being off the workaday calendar—though those things seem plausible, too. Given how a young Jew of his time would have felt about the Sabbath, you can't help but suspect that the boy would have had to fight his way to his family's Friday-night dinner table through a storm of emotions: the disgust felt when your parents practice rites you deem primitive; the guilt inspired by such disgust; the alienation you feel when you don't know whether to be loyal to your family or to the outside world. No wonder he threw up. No wonder he found himself on Ferenczi's couch. The question is why Ferenczi, who must have had firsthand experience with the same internal Kulturkampf, never entertains the possibility that the Sabbath itself (rather than Sabbath-related sexual activities) could have been the source of the boy's distress—or at least Ferenczi never utters the thought. But maybe the mental picture of a Sabbath table made Ferenczi a little queasy himself.

5.
—

It wasn't just the times that changed in the shift from Ferenczi's parents' generation to his, or from my grandparents' to mine. Time changed, too. We tend to forget that time itself has a history. Consider that only thirty-five years before Ferenczi's essay, twenty-five nations in Europe and the Americas began the process of unifying all the local times around the globe into a single mesh of standard public time, dissecting the world into twenty-four time zones, with Greenwich, England, as the zero meridian. Not coincidentally, at the same point in history artists and writers were beginning to chronicle the rise of the diametrically opposite kind of time: idiosyncratic private time. Psychological man defined himself in opposition to the clock. In *The Culture of Time and Space: 1880–1918,* the cultural historian Stephen Kern proves this point by riffling through the works of the great turn-of-the-century chroniclers of consciousness: the philosopher Henri Bergson, the psychologist William James, Marcel Proust, James Joyce, Franz Kafka, and, of course, Freud. Kafka wrote: "It's impossible to sleep, impossible to wake, impossible to bear life or, more precisely, the successiveness of life. The clocks don't agree. The inner one rushes along in a devilish or demonic—in any case, inhuman—way while the outer one goes, falteringly, its accustomed pace." Freud, ever the encyclopedist, saw that private time could sometimes be swift, sometimes be slow. Dreams turned the plodding sequences of waking life into rapid-fire montage, but the unconscious could move with glacial indifference to ordinary standards of time.

Taken together as a dialectical unit, however, private and public time were eclipsing an older kind of time: religious time. Ferenczi may have elevated the Christian calendar, with its Sundays, to the public standard of all civilization, but by the early twentieth century factories and department stores were no longer uniformly closing on Sundays, and Christians were beginning to grasp what it meant to worship as a minority (and were beginning to complain about it). Public time was time calibrated to the needs of transportation and production networks. Private time was equally desacralized and irreligious. Sacred calendars were—and are—sternly communitarian. Religious time does not strive to satisfy individual needs. It makes its own inexorable demands, flowing from prayer service to prayer service, from festival to festival.

For men and women—or boys and girls—as determinedly forward-looking as Ferenczi and his patients were, religious time must have seemed vertiginously de trop. Think of sacred holidays as wells; they tunnel down through temporal strata and allow the past to bubble into the present through the liquid medium of myth. Keeping the Sabbath means sliding the cover off that hole on a weekly basis. It is easy to imagine a turn-of-the-century youth peering into the *mise en abyme* of time past that is the Sabbath and feeling sort of sick.

6.
___

IN FERENCZI'S DAY, it was communitarian time that seemed on the verge of disappearing. Now family time does, too. Not long ago, the sociologist Arlie Hochschild studied life at Amerco, an unusually worker-friendly Fortune 500 company. In her 1997 book *The Time Bind,* she reported that workers had grown so entranced with life in their workplace that they'd started avoiding their less well-tended-to personal lives. To maximize the time spent in the office or on take-home work, they applied managerial principles of efficiency to their homes and their children. The faster the Amerco employee got through the dishes, the sooner she could get back to work.

Today, work has grown even more portable, so that the work addict need never turn off her mobile communications device as she interacts with her family. This image of the workaholic may be a caricature, but caricatures only exaggerate the satirizable features of everyday life. And if there's one thing we know about everyday life, it's that we don't have enough time to finish our work and get our chores done and be with family and friends.

We don't actually work more than we used to, but we think we do. In 1991, the economist Juliet Schor advanced the now conventional thesis that global competition forced Americans to toil longer and rest less. She based this on rough estimates that people gave during interviews with U.S. census takers over three decades. Meanwhile, two sociologists, John P. Robinson and Geoffrey Godbey, were asking people to fill out time diaries noting exactly how much time they spent on each activity of the day right after they'd done it. They concluded that Americans work less than they did in the 1960s. How do you reconcile what people said with what their time diaries showed? You acknowledge that Americans *feel* more pressed for time, whether they're working harder or not.

Many theories have been advanced to explain the perception that we're overtaxed. Some cite evidence that it's mainly highly educated white-collar workers who put in those legendary fifty-, sixty-, seventy-hour weeks, even as blue-collar or service workers struggle to cobble together enough work to live on. Others interpret our feeling of being overwhelmed as a function of the fact that, even though as employees we work no more than we used to, as family members more of us are saddled with more of the burdens of domestic life. The women who used to stay home and take care of everything now leave their houses for offices, so that chores must be more evenly distributed throughout the family. People have that nagging sense of never having finished with the housework, even though if you added up all the hours we collectively devote to housework, you'd find that the number is smaller than it was thirty years ago (down from slightly more than twenty-seven hours a week to twenty-four).

Time *has* become more fragmented. More Americans work during the off-hours than they did half a century ago, the heyday of the nine-to-five, Monday-through-Friday workweek. According to the sociologist Harriet B. Presser, as of 2003, two-fifths of American workers were working non-standard hours—"in the evening, at night, on a rotating shift, or during the weekend"—and she wasn't counting those who bring their work home and do it on their off-hours, or who are self-employed. Some people have enviable flexibility. They've won flextime from their bosses, hold non-traditional jobs, or are self-employed. Others have no choice but to work late shifts at companies that measure time by overseas clocks, or else they've found employment in the service sector, to which the bulk of American jobs have shifted. There they wait on everybody else in the evenings and on weekends.

Shift work, it is now clear, disrupts circadian rhythms, fosters insomnia, and induces inattentiveness, memory loss, and depression, especially when the shifts are irregular. This is because different parts of the body's ecosystem—temperature, hormones, the heart, the digestive system—adjust to disrupted sleep schedules at different rates, causing parts of the body to be at war with others. Flextime workers don't have the same physical problems, but their irregular work hours nonetheless upset their psychological equilibrium. With a moment snatched here and there, it's hard to achieve that feeling of being in the swing of something, the self-forgetfulness that psychologists call flow. Moreover, when friends and family no longer follow the same schedule they're less likely to get together. According to Presser, couples who have children and work separate shifts are more likely to get divorced than those who don't—as much as six times as likely when it's the husband who works the late-night shift, or on a rotating schedule, and three times as likely when it's the wife.

But we tend not to see these problems as the result of living in a temporally discombobulated society. We blame ourselves. We say that we're too busy to do everything we want to do and see the people we want to see, and isn't that a shame. Besides, even if we aren't working more than we used to, we don't get as much done during our non-work hours as we wish we did. The time-diary studies suggest that we feel as if we're falling short because we devote just under half of our free time to media: at the time of the study, mostly television; to a lesser degree newspapers, radio, and books; and now, one assumes, iPhones, computer games, and the Web. And though we squander more hours on television and computers, we ask more of ourselves in the hours remaining. We try to train ourselves to use our free time more efficiently: to master more kinds of time-saving technology; to become more proficient skiers or chess players or home decorators; to maximize face time with our loved ones; to live up to ecological mandates for a more handcrafted domestic life.

7.

WHAT IS HAPPENING to us? Nothing to get worked up about. This is life in an industrial and postindustrial and post-postindustrial society. "The clock, not the steam-engine, is the key-machine of the modern industrial age," Lewis Mumford wrote. Ever since the early fourteenth century, when Italian churchmen and city fathers began adorning their towers with publicly visible clocks, we have been governed by increasingly precise instruments of time measurement. It was public clocks, then household clocks, then watches, then stopwatches, and, ultimately, the atomic clock, that made it possible to coordinate and schedule more and more complex networks of manufacturing, labor, and trade.

One weirdly delightful fact about clocks is that they made possible a new crime: time theft. According to the British social historian E. P. Thompson, eighteenth- and nineteenth-century masters and managers stole time from their workers. They put the factories' clocks forward in the morning and back at night, so that workers had to come in earlier and leave later without being paid for more work. One English worker told an investigating committee about a clock with a weighted minute hand that, as soon as it started on its downward slope, dropped three minutes at a time. It was used to shorten the dinner hour. Time was money, as Benjamin Franklin said, and had to be made to pay. The sharp use of time became the moral obligation of the businessman. "The infraction of its rules is treated not as foolishness but as forgetfulness of duty," Max Weber declared in *The Protestant Ethic and the Spirit of Capitalism*.

Two giants of temporal thrift, Frederick Winslow Taylor and Henry Ford, pushed us into the modern era at the turn of the twen-

tieth century. Taylor invented time-and-motion studies. Ford stan-
dardized and quickened production by breaking down tasks for the
assembly line. Postwar "post-Fordism" brought, among other things,
"vertical disintegration"—subcontracting and outsourcing—as well
as small-batch and just-in-time and globally networked production,
electronic banking, computerized trading, and the more rapid pace of
consumption that follows from a switch from a commodity-based to
a service-based economy. (It takes less time to see a movie than to
wear out a coat.)

It wasn't until the second half of the twentieth century that anyone noticed that all this time-saving didn't make us feel less rushed.
On the contrary. "We had always expected one of the beneficent results of economic affluence to be a tranquil and harmonious manner
of life, a life in Arcadia," the Swedish economist Staffan Linder wrote
in his 1970 book *The Harried Leisure Class.* "What has happened is the
exact opposite. The pace is quickening, and our lives in fact are becoming more hectic." Linder's theory was that as labor becomes more
specialized and productivity increases, two things happen. First, each
hour of work increases in value, which jacks up the value of hours
spent not working. Non-work time has a higher "opportunity
cost"—each minute not spent completing one's work assignments
equals more money squandered. Second, there are ever more products
to consume.

Linder realized that these outcomes cancel each other out. He
was the first to point out something that has since become obvious:
To calculate the real cost of consumption, you have to factor in the
real amount of time spent consuming. Consuming is not just buying.
Not only do we need time to make smart decisions about our new
cars, high-definition televisions, and lawn mowers; we also need time
to read the instruction manuals or call the help desk in order to learn
to use all our increasingly complicated gadgets. And we need to keep
them in good shape or get them repaired. In short, as time becomes
more valuable to us, our consumer goods become more expensive
to us.

One solution to the problem of maintenance is to outsource it. In the decades since Linder's book, outsourcing has expanded to include not just the upkeep and the repairs we used to do ourselves (laundry, lawn work, home repair, child care) but chores and roles once considered too personal or trivial to hire someone to do, from organizing garages to filling in at social occasions for the spouses we don't have time to court and marry. From a financial point of view, though, outsourcing is not the answer. The price of personal services rises as more people buy them, which means those same people have to work more to foot the monthly bill for their in-house or subcontracted support staffs. The grueling hours endured by handsomely paid professionals, it turns out, don't necessarily reflect work addiction. Putting in those hours may be the only way to stay ahead of the bill collector.

The other solution to the time famine is to cram more activities into the same span of time. Not long after Linder's book appeared, Erwin Scheuch, a German sociologist who had conducted a time-diary study in twelve countries, noticed that the more industrialized the country, the more likely a person was to crowd more activities into the same twenty-four hours. Scheuch called this "time-deepening," by analogy to the economic concept of "capital deepening"—getting the same output from a production process at a lower cost.

Time-deepening spares our pocketbooks, even if it reduces the intensity of our pleasure. In that sense, Scheuch's phrase is misleading, because stuffing life with more things and distractions makes time feel shallower, not deeper. "Time-stretching" may be a better term. Whatever you call it, Linder accurately predicted how it would affect the texture of our lives. He anticipated the rising preference for fast food, quickie sex, drive-through banking, and so on, as well as the predictable rejection of such things by those élite contrarians who could afford slow food, old-fashioned courtship, and personal bankers.

Linder also foresaw subtler impacts. Lacking the leisure to research all the goods and services that we feel compelled to purchase, we rely more and more on what Linder calls "ersatz information," or advertising, which lets people feel they're still getting enough input to make a good decision. (Linder wrote his book before the explosion of "branding," but he would have seen brand identification as yet another form of overreliance on ersatz information.)

Home is the place where we dream of escaping the time-and-motion calculus. Family time is best measured by the activity, not by the clock. You serve your stew when it's ready, not when it has cooked for an hour. You put away your sponges and cleaning fluids when your bathroom is clean, not after five minutes. You nurse a baby until she's full, whether that takes ten minutes or forty. This form of time measurement is known as task orientation, and it is the kind of time that is kept in less industrialized societies. Task orientation is also characterized by a tendency not to make overly fine distinctions between "work" (doing chores) and "life" (chatting, eating, relaxing).

People used to working a set number of hours often find the task-oriented approach to time scandalously wasteful, an attitude that can contribute to misunderstandings not only between industrialized and non-industrialized cultures but also between spouses, especially when one works out of the home and the other stays in it. "Despite school times and television times, the rhythms of women's work in the home are not wholly attuned to the measurement of the clock," E. P. Thompson wrote. "The mother of young children has an imperfect sense of time and attends to other human tides. She has not yet altogether moved out of the conventions of 'pre-industrial' time."

But time in the home is still money. Feminist economics has taught us that the domestic sphere floated above the sordid dominion of the dollar only because it relied on the free labor and the forgone opportunities of women. Ever since women grew weary of the unwritten rule deeming their time worth what they were paid for it, it has gotten harder to find anyone—Linder would say, to pay anyone enough—to invest the time to meet our most intimate physical and emotional needs.

We all know what it feels like to give short shrift to ourselves, our families, and our children, not to mention the stranger in our midst. It feels disgusting. Our bodies, our houses, and our relationships spiral toward disorder and decay. Our nails lengthen because we forget to cut them. Our eyesight blurs because we can't be bothered to visit the eye doctor. Slime accumulates on pantry shelves. The tone in our spouses' voices hardens. Children mutiny at times seemingly calculated to be inconvenient. Too busy to attend to our own needs, we lack sympathy for the needs of people who seem less busy than we are. That, too, has consequences. Before long, the underemployed become the unemployable, then the menacing mob.

8.

THE SABBATH—God's claim against our time—implies that time has an ethical dimension. We rest in order to honor God and his creation, which suggests that not to rest dishonors both. So must we say that the speeding up of everything is not only psychologically harmful but *morally* wrong? What about the contravening benefits of super-productivity—the wealth, health, democracy, and philanthropy that come with it?

In 1973, the social psychologists John Darley and Daniel Batson performed an experiment that was meant to explore a dimension of the human personality, but along the way they stumbled onto something important about the ethics of time. Their question was, What makes a passerby decide whether to stop to help someone in distress? Is it personality, cultural conditioning, or the situation at hand? Darley and Batson wanted to know which of these variables had the greatest influence on whether a person acted like the Good Samaritan in Jesus' parable of that name:

A certain man went down from Jerusalem to Jericho, and fell among thieves, which stripped him of his raiment, and wounded him, and departed, leaving him half dead. And by chance there came down a certain priest that way: and when he saw him, he passed by on the other side. And likewise a Levite, when he was at the place, came and looked on him, and passed by on the other side. But a certain Samaritan, as he journeyed, came where he was: and when he saw him, he had compassion on him, and went to him, and bound up his wounds, pouring in oil and wine, and set him on his own beast, and brought him to an inn, and took care of him. And on the morrow when he departed, he took out two pence, and gave them to the host, and said unto him, Take care of him; and whatsoever thou spendest more, when I come again, I will repay thee.

Looking for test subjects who were likely to have made the message of the parable a part of their lives, Darley and Batson recruited students from the Princeton Theological Seminary. Their study proceeded as follows: First, the researchers ran tests to determine each student's personality type. Then the researchers announced that they needed more information. The students would have to give a talk. Half of them were asked to deliver a sermon on the Good Samaritan. The other half were told to discuss the job prospects that faced them as future ministers and were instructed to report to another building, where their audiences would be waiting for them. As the students left the first building, a researcher urged about a third of them to hurry, because they were already late. He assured another third that they were right on time but shouldn't dawdle. He told the last third that there was a slight delay in the proceedings but that they should wander over anyway. As the students walked to the second building, they passed a man slumped against a doorway in an alley. They didn't know it, but this was the real test. As each student approached, the man coughed and groaned. If the student stopped, the man told them in a confused and groggy voice that he was fine but he had a respiratory condition; he had taken medicine that would begin to work any minute now. If the student insisted on helping the man, he allowed himself to be taken into a building nearby.

After the data was weighted and the variables analyzed, only one variable could be used to predict who would stop to help and who wouldn't. The important factor was not personality type or whether a student's career or the parable of the Good Samaritan was fo___ ___st in his mind. It was whether or not he was in a hurry. Person___ significance only among those students who stopped. Partic___ pathetic students stayed with the man longer; those who ___

nally rigid forced him to drink a glass of water even when he said he didn't want one. As for the effects of culture, Darley and Batson pointed out that it would be hard to name a cultural norm more powerful for a seminary student than the example of the Good Samaritan, but it still didn't make a student more likely to stop.

The study made it hard not to conclude, said Darley and Batson, "that ethics becomes a luxury as the speed of our daily lives increases." The psychologists weren't quick to judge these seminarians. Even though all the students who hadn't stopped admitted that they'd seen the man, Darley and Batson pointed out, several said that they hadn't realized that he needed help until after they'd passed him. Time pressure had narrowed their "cognitive map"; as they raced by they had seen without seeing.

Meanwhile, the students who had realized that the man required assistance but had withheld it from him showed up for their talks looking "aroused and anxious." Darley and Batson speculated that their subjects felt torn between their duty to help the man and their desire to live up to the expectations of the psychologists whose test they had freely agreed to take. "This is often true of people in a hurry," Darley and Batson wrote. "They hurry because somebody depends on their being somewhere. Conflict, rather than callousness, can explain their failure to stop."

9.

THE ONE THING I DO CONSISTENTLY on Friday nights is drink, I drink whether I'm at home or at a more traditionally laid Sabbath table or attending an entirely non-Jewish event that I couldn't bring myself to pass up. I drink red wine, if I can, and right up to the line where looseness looks a lot like rudeness. Preferring not to think of myself as a weekly alcoholic, I tell myself that wine stands in for the Sabbaths I so rarely manage to keep. A full-bodied red wine is what a poet might call the objective correlative of the Sabbath, with the color of kosher wine I sipped as a child (though not the poisonous sweetness), the warmth of the candles, the mollifying effect on critical consciousness that Ferenczi said Sunday ought to have.

This is not precisely in the spirit of the Jewish Sabbath, but there is a family resemblance to it. The rabbis disapproved of drunkenness, but they also decreed that the Sabbath be a time for joy. "Call the Sabbath a delight," the prophet Isaiah said. Not being nearly as impractical as they are often made out to have been, the rabbis knew that you couldn't rejoice without good food and strong drink. "When the Holy Temple stood, there was no rejoicing without meat," the Talmud says. "Now that the Holy Temple is not standing, there is no rejoicing without wine." Note the logic of substitution at work in that saying: We ate meat when we brought sacrifices to the Temple, but now that there's no Temple we drink wine. Religions evolve through a process of condensation—call it distillation. First there's some primal spiritual experience, then it's boiled down to a symbol; when the old symbol threatens to lose its power, we turn up the heat to intensify it. Jesus was fortifying an ancient symbol with a strong new spirit when he told his disciples at the Last Supper, "This cup is the new testament in my blood."

Sometimes I think that drinking wine is the only form of religiosity I can consistently muster. This is slightly less crazy than it sounds. There's an old habit in religious life of achieving joy by oenophilic means. Everyone swigs wine in the Bible, and a social historian named Elliott Horowitz has collected a remarkably large number of examples of ancient, medieval, and early-modern Jews pushing the Sabbath delights—drinking, copulating, and schmoozing—a lot further than you'd expect them to, at least if you're foolish enough to believe the usual clichés about Jews being sober and law-abiding. In the first century, Plutarch speculated that the Jews had a Dionysian streak, since they were so eager to celebrate the Sabbath by urging drink on one another. Horowitz recounts tales of Sabbath drinking contests held by fifteenth-century Egyptian Jews; he tells of a seventeenth-century rabbi in Frankfurt who chided the young men of his synagogue for drinking brandy during the Saturday-morning service, "sometimes becoming so drunk they forgot to recite the musaf prayer." The repetitive songs sung at the close of the Passover service—the Seder, in which one is expected to drink at least four cups of wine—are said to derive from nursery songs, but they also have the classic structure of drinking songs: the repeated refrains, the lengthening verses, the fixed rhythms, the simple lyrics. The same can be said of many of the songs sung—or, rather, roared—after dinner around a Sabbath table. "Work makes for prosperous days; wine makes for happy Sundays," as Charles Baudelaire put it in an essay on wine and hashish. Wine is the Sabbath in a bottle. Wine steps in when religion loses force.

Rarely, if ever, do Americans encounter the so-called blue laws once enforced in most states, banning all behavior deemed non-Sabbath-like—everything from traveling to card-playing and pawn-broking. But when we do it's usually because a checkout clerk in a grocery store has refused to sell us beer or wine before noon on Sunday. You can deduce that drinking was the norm on British Sundays from these Puritan bans on alcohol, which were never fully enforced, not even in the seventeenth century, at the height of Puritan power. Puritan efforts to legislate Sunday drinking out of existence have left on the record a pungent portrait of the raucous Sundays common when the laws were written. The Sunday Law enacted under King James VI in 1656 reads:

> Every person being in any Tavern, Inn, Alehouse, Victualling house, Strongwater house, Tobacco house, Celler or Shop, . . . or fetching or sending for any wine, ale, or beer, tobacco, strongwater, or other strong liquor unnecessarily, and to tipple within any other house or shop; . . . and every common brewer and baker, brewing and baking, or causing bread to be baked, or beer and ale to be brewed upon the day aforesaid. . . . All persons keeping, using, or being present upon the day aforesaid at any Fairs, Markets, Wakes, Revels, Wrestling, Shootings, Leaping, Bowling, Ringing of Bells for pleasure, or upon any other occasion (save for calling people together for the public

Worship), Feasts, Church Ale, May-Poles, Gaming, Bear-baiting, Bull-Baiting, or any other Sports and Pastimes . . . shall be deemed guilty of profaning the Lord's Day.

On Friday nights, when I lived in the suburbs, I had at least one glass of wine before putting my two children in the car and driving to services. If you looked at the synagogue I was driving to, a tiny congregation in a big dilapidated house in a relatively Christian town, you would wonder why a woman would jeopardize her children's lives to get there. The sanctuary was dark and homely. The wool on its kitschy Israeli wall hangings had begun to ball up. The services were sparsely attended by suburbanites in sweatpants or jeans. The tunes were tuneless—more like chanting—though hypnotic over time. If you could read the liturgy in Hebrew, its outrageous grandeur would make you forget the irritation you might naturally feel at being forced to read poetry before dinner at the end of a hard week. But if you couldn't you were stuck reading translations that flattened magnificence into an institutionalized vision of exaltation.

But I liked standing in a room singing with a group of people I may not always have considered intimate friends but was glad to see once a week. Many of them seemed slightly drunk themselves, or maybe they were just getting ready to be. They swept my children up into bear hugs. They made room for us in the back. The children dashed out into the hall as soon as I let them, so that they could run up and down it with their playmates. The adults clapped and swayed awkwardly, with middle-aged bodies no longer adept at spontaneous movement.

Some would call this community. I like the anthropologist Victor Turner's word, "communitas." He was talking about the kind of group life that emerges at the edges of society, not in the middle of it, where people search for something—meaning, solace, truths—that the larger society doesn't seem to offer. *Communitas* describes a gathering that may be a little offbeat, a little decrepit, rather hard to see the point of if you're peering in from outside. Communitas is what happened in the services in private homes that early Christians attended, where they broke the bread and drank the wine and spun out in ever more mythologized detail the stories that would eventually become the Gospels. Communitas, in its common focus on an ideal or a dream, is non-hierarchical and anti-institutional and intoxicating and intimate and also strangely, frighteningly impersonal. Under the spell of a charismatic tyrant, a Mao or a Stalin, communitas can yield the lawless ethos of a mob. Martin Buber meant communitas when he wrote: "Community is the being no longer side by side (and, one might add, above and below) but *with* one another of a multitude of persons. And this multitude, though it moves toward one goal, yet experiences everywhere a turning to, a dynamic facing of, the others, a flowing from *I* to *Thou*." Communitas is the beginning of a shadow of a very old idea of the Sabbath.

PART TWO

GROUP DYNAMICS

1.

IF WE ARE TO FEEL OUR WAY INTO THE PSYCHES OF THE MEN AND women who held the Sabbath so dear that they made it the Fourth Commandment—placing it above the injunction against murder—we have to start with the sensation of heat: scorching, air-conditioner-less, soul-withering heat. It is the hot part of the summer in a small city in a tiny desert nation in the 586th year before the advent of the Christian era. The Babylonian king Nebuchadnezzar has been canni-balizing an empire from the aging parts of previous ones in Assyria and Egypt. Eleven years earlier, he had punished a rebellious king of the state of Judah by laying siege to its capital, Jerusalem, and exiling said king, along with several thousand of the nation's leading citizens and craftsmen. A Babylonian puppet had been put on the throne, but the puppet had rebelled as well, and now Nebuchadnezzar's army was once again at the walls of the city. The Babylonian soldiers had built siege towers and mounds and hunkered down. They had let neither water nor food into the city, and no one was allowed to leave. The corpses of the parched and the starved lay scattered in the streets, and no one still alive had the wherewithal to fight off the men in glinting helmets who were about to pour in through the breaches they had just made in the walls.

It is considered credulous to take biblical poetry as literal truth, but when it comes to the siege of Jerusalem there are several accounts written early enough after the city's sacking and the destruction of its Temple to offer eyewitness testimony. The book of Lamentations, in particular, brings a specificity to its itemization of horror that gives it the force of documentary. "The emotion seems too raw for a poem," the poet and Bible translator Stephen Mitchell has said of Lamentations. "The reality is too raw." Skeptical archaeologists have not yet managed to contradict the biblical account of famine. On the contrary, some fecal remains found in a toilet in use at the time support its historical accuracy, revealing a diet light on nutrients and heavy on roadside weeds and the kinds of parasites that enter the stomach through rotting meat. Lamentations fills in the details. "The tongue of the suckling [child] cleaves to its palate for thirst," the poet writes. (Because they convey the graphic concreteness of Lamentations with particular faithfulness, the translations given from that book come from the Jewish Publication Society edition of the Hebrew Bible. All other biblical citations in the book come from the King James Version, by far the greater work of literature.) "Those who feasted on dainties lie famished in the streets; those who were reared in purple have embraced refuse heaps." (The King James Bible translates this, more bluntly, as "lie in dunghills.") "Alas, women eat their own fruit, their new-born babes!"

On the day that the Babylonians breached the wall, say the authors of the biblical histories known as First and Second Kings, they established a base at one of Jerusalem's main gates but didn't enter the palace. That night, Judah's king, Zedekiah, and his soldiers and family sneaked out of the city through the palace garden and fled toward the Jordan. "But the Babylonian troops pursued the king," we read in Second Kings, "and they overtook him in the steppes of Jericho as his entire force left him and scattered. They captured the king and brought him before the king of Babylon at Riblah; and they put him on trial."

Nebuchadnezzar had his officials kill Zedekiah's sons in front of him, put his eyes out, chain him up, and take him to Babylon.

The prophet Jeremiah adds that the king of Babylon "slew all the nobles of Judah," too. Then Nebuchadnezzar's troops set fire to Jerusalem, tore down its walls, and sacked the Temple, carrying off anything made of bronze, silver, or gold. They killed everyone who got in their way, rounded up the survivors, and marched them into exile, though not before singling out several top officials and sixty commoners for execution. Only the "poorest in the land" were allowed to remain, to be "vinedressers and field hands."

The Babylonian exile may be the most bitterly objected-to population transfer in all Western literature. Several of the later books in the Hebrew Bible dwell upon it with obsessive anguish, interpreting it self-laceratingly as God's punishment of an insubordinate people. Many books—such as Exodus, with its tales of enslavement, and Deuteronomy, with its concern for the well-being of servants—have been interpreted as allegories of the experience, quasi-historical novels making an unbearable present palatable by setting it in the past. In every case in which the exile is discussed directly, rather than obliquely, the language is as skinless as meat. What does it mean to be starved, dehydrated, conquered, and deported? It is, say the poets, like being gang-raped: "The foe has laid hands on everything dear to her" ("her" is Jerusalem); "she has seen her Sanctuary invaded by nations." It is like being forced into prostitution, then made to walk down a public thoroughfare in whore's clothing: "All who admired her despise her, for they have seen her disgraced; and she can only sigh and shrink back. Her uncleanness clings to her skirts." It is like having one's father bash one's head against the pavement: "He"—meaning God—"has broken my teeth on gravel, has ground me into the dust."

It was out of this abasement that Judaism as we know it was born, and along with it the Sabbath.

2.

THIS IS NOT TO SAY that the religion of the Bible, including the Sabbath, hadn't existed before the exile. Clearly, it had, for hundreds of years. By the time the Babylonians carried off the Israelite priests, the form of worship they helped their people conduct was well established, though its origins and its earliest history remain mysterious.

The Sabbath was at least as old as the cult itself, if not older, although, again, no one knows how old *old* is, and whether the Sabbath was kept in a strict fashion or not, or exactly what keeping it would have entailed. Resting on the seventh day may initially have been no more than an accidentally savvy social arrangement—the wise management of land and human resources in an early, fragile agricultural society—and only later acquired theological connotations. (Two Sabbath-like land- and debt-management customs codified in the Bible—the sabbatical year and the jubilee year—suggest this origin. The sabbatical occurs every seventh year. During that year, farmers must leave their land fallow and all outstanding debts between Israelites must be canceled. The jubilee occurs every fifty years, on the year following seven sabbaticals. During a jubilee year, the laws of the sabbatical must be observed, but two more rules apply as well: All hereditary land must revert to its original owners or their heirs, and all Hebrew slaves, who were likely to have sold themselves into slavery to pay off their debts, must be freed.) Or the Sabbath may have expressed a taboo, a fear of arousing the wrath of an irascible god. The Sabbath may have been one of Israel's festivals, a day of joyous feasting much like the day of the new moon. (Some have theorized that it was once the day of the full moon.) It may have been part of the popular religion, observed mainly through sacrifices in family compounds. Or it may have been a priestly matter involving formal Temple sacrifices. It's even possible that the ancient Sabbath looked a lot more like the modern one than we have any right to expect. Already in the eighth century B.C.E.—two centuries before the exile—a prophet, Amos, sounds remarkably like a modern clergyman when he chides his people for tolerating merchants who are too greedy to wait for the end of the Sabbath to start selling their wares.

But all of these are speculations, because the prehistory of the Sabbath is just that: that which occurred before the histories were written. There is little physical evidence for the Sabbath outside the Bible. Nor can we compare it with similar institutions in the cultures that surrounded the spit of land that became the twin states of Israel and Judah, because, oddly enough, the Sabbath appears to have been the invention of the inhabitants of those two tiny nations. Many scholars have tried to link the Hebrew Sabbath to some analogous non-Hebrew practice, but their theories have turned out to be implausible or unprovable. There is some charm to the theory that the weekly day of non-work, whose most stringent prohibition forbade the lighting of fires, derived from the fire taboo of a tribe called the Kenites, said to have been blacksmiths and worshippers of Saturn. This hypothesis "is both ingenious and fragile," as one scholar writes, because we have almost no information about the Kenites, other than that they lived in the Sinai; we don't know "whether they really were blacksmiths, or whether they knew of the week, or whether they venerated Saturn."

The evocative similarity of the Hebrew word *Shabbat* to an ancient Akkadian word, *shappatu,* the day of the full moon, an auspicious day "when the gods' heart was appeased," has tantalized many and probably has some relevance, but no one can quite say how much. So does the likeness of the Hebrew Sabbath to the Babylonian *ume lemnuti,* evil or inauspicious days, which fell on the seventh, fourteenth, twenty-first, and twenty-eighth day of the month (and possibly also the nineteenth), and on which, according to the ancient texts, "the shepherd of the peoples [that is, the king] must not eat cooked meat or baked bread, must not change his clothes or put on clean clothes, must not offer sacrifice, must not go out in his chariot or exercise his sovereign power. The priest must not deliver oracles, and the physician must not touch the sick. It is an unsuitable day for any kind of action."

Suggestive as they may be, the *ume lemnuti* fall short of Sabbaths in many ways. For one thing, the Hebrew Sabbath required the participation of all the people, not just the king. Moreover, the Sabbath, which comes every seventh day regardless of the length of the month, was not grounded in the lunar calendar. It was severed from the phases of the moon, if it had ever been yoked to them.

This lack of clear answers leaves us dissatisfied. When we go hunting for origins, we want objects, documents, dates, stones with worn inscriptions. We want to conjure up the archaeological dig in which proof of the Sabbath would have been waved triumphantly aloft. But the Sabbath is a ritual, not an artifact. It is not an object built in space; it is a performance enacted in time. What we do know is that it was during the Israelites' sojourn in Mesopotamia and in the decades after, when a Persian king named Cyrus conquered the Babylonians and, incredibly, sent the exiles back to rebuild their land, that the Israelites began to collect their folktales and their legal and theological traditions and weave them into a book: the Hebrew Bible.

If we want to look to the Bible to understand how our ancestors felt about the Sabbath, we have to remember that while the Bible teaches us our history, it is not history in any sense that we've ever been taught. Nor is it literature, exactly. It's both and neither, a strange amalgam of prose and poetry, containing scene after scene of some of the most profound drama conceived by the cosmological imagination. Does the Bible tell of things as they were, elevating actual occurrences to a mythological plane? Or does it consist of brilliant imaginings, taut parables craftily distressed by some unknown genius to exhibit the grit and anguish of history? Is there a meaningful difference? "For a people in ancient times these were legitimate and sometimes inevitable modes of historical perception and interpretation," Yerushalmi writes. Émile Durkheim invented the sociology of religion in the early part of the twentieth century by making the still controversial claim that religions "are grounded in and express the real," by which he meant the reality of a collective or social experience. But, he added, "although religious thought is something other than a system of fictions, the realities to which it corresponds can gain religious expression only if imagination transfigures them."

The priests who wrote the Bible did so for many reasons, but one of the most important was to preserve and revive a way of life and a worldview that, for all they knew, was about to disappear from the earth. And so it is as a response to exile that we must seek the meanings of the day itself.

3.
—

IF I WERE FORCED to single out one thing that is truly exceptional about the Sabbath, it would have to be its efficacy. The Sabbath *does* something, and what it does is remarkable. People who study the ways in which cultures evolve might say that the Sabbath gives societies a competitive advantage. It promotes social solidarity.

Imagine that there was a job called "social architect," and you had it. Your job description would be dreaming up the perfect society, drafting the blueprint for it, overseeing its construction from scratch. (In real life, of course, this job is relatively rare, and to the degree that it exists it's generally unpopular. The past century has provided ample evidence that social engineering, at least on a large scale, tends to end in tragedy or atrocity.) Casting around for existing social institutions to model your new society on, you'd happen upon the Sabbath. If a strong and powerfully interconnected communal life was high on your priority list, you'd quickly realize that you had stumbled on a very good way to achieve it, because the Sabbath can easily be reconfigured as a four-step program for forging community spirit.

In the first step, you'd write laws to limit work time. That would make room for other kinds of time—rest time, recreational time, family time, time for friends and guests, and, of course, time for God. In the second step, you'd designate one particular day as everybody's day off. That would coordinate schedules, so that people across a wide range of occupations and social spheres would all have to stop working at the same time and be forced to turn toward one another, individually and in groups. The third step would be to ordain that the day off be taken every single week, rather than now and again, so that not working at that time would become a regular habit. Once the weekly rhythm of work and rest had become ingrained, it would set your community apart; it would establish clear boundaries between your society and all others, and boundaries, as everyone knows, are wonderful tools for ensuring the cohesiveness of a group. And fourth, you'd make the day festive, filled with song, wine, food, and pretty clothes. People would come to look forward to the day as a treat, rather than experiencing its restrictions as a burden.

Laws that limit time, coordinate schedules, force people to make a habit of getting together at a prescribed time—all this strikes us as un-American. Besides, life today forbids it. Our wealth as a nation depends on a delicately interlaced network of flexible schedules, our ability to differentiate among kinds of labor and perform them in the proper sequence. Who would want to do without the industries that manufacture products sporadically and in a rush, whenever there's a demand for them? What about factories whose equipment is so expensive they must operate 24/7? Or the artists and loners who thrive on their weird schedules, and need restaurants and bars with matching weird schedules, and who generate the new ideas that push us forward into the future?

In a study of the American laws that govern time, the Harvard law professor Todd D. Rakoff asks us to imagine a world divided between two completely opposed kinds of regimes, a "freedom of time regime" and a "constructed time regime." In the freedom-of-time regime, people dispose of their time as they see fit, and the law does nothing more than lay down and enforce the conditions under which individuals and institutions get to swap time for money. I may work for you for as many hours a week as you'll pay me for, and at whatever times we both agree on, and only if one of us breaks his side of the bargain does anyone go to court. In the constructed-time regime, the law designates a certain period of time as social time, or at least mandates that some amount of time may not be work time. Rakoff's prime example of constructed-time lawmaking is, in fact, the Sabbath, as exemplified by America's now mostly defunct blue, or Sunday-closing, laws: "six-sevenths commercial time and one-seventh noncommercial (family, religious, or social) time." (The Fair Labor Standards Act reflects a more minimalist constructed-time ideology, since it mandates overtime when a wage earner works more than forty hours. Under the FLSA, I'm required to work for you for only, say, forty hours a week, unless you pay me a whole lot more. With blue laws, you couldn't pay me to work on Sunday, even if we both wanted me to.)

The freedom-of-time approach sounds right to us, because we think of time as money, which is to say, a fungible resource. Anything that gets in the way of our freely allocating our time doesn't just get on our nerves; it prevents us from coming up with the most efficient way of using our time. In the language of the marketplace, it's irrational. "If, for example, a society forbade all night work," Rakoff says, "that would prevent firms from doing at night things which are best segregated from the work of the day; the very fact that without the prohibition there would be night work serves as proof . . . that there is such work worth doing." The usual objection to a system based purely on individual contracts is that there's some imbalance of power between the parties making them, which means that one side isn't quite as free as the other. That's easily corrected; all you have to do is craft some narrowly worded law that forbids this or that form of coercion, and voilà! Your market is operating more rationally than ever before.

But there's a flaw in the main assumption of the freedom-of-time regime: that time is, like money, a pure quantity to be divided and spent at will. One minute is not exactly like every other minute, because time changes as it flows. Time is qualitative as well as quantitative. The *when* of time—its *after what* or *before what* or *at the same time as what*—matters as much as, if not more than, its *how much*. It makes a big difference whether you do something now or wait till later. We know all this intuitively, because we would have no social or professional lives if we didn't.

To borrow one of Eviatar Zerubavel's examples, sex means one thing on the first date and something else altogether on the twenti-eth. Fifteen minutes matters a great deal when you're late for a sales call, but counts for almost nothing when you're waltzing into a cock-tail party. The value of time is relative and situational. The true cost of a minute can't be calculated unless you factor in who is doing what when and with whom. One hour spent listening to the leading thinkers on housing policy is worth at least as much, to the head of Housing and Urban Development, as the several hours he spent set-ting up the panel and wooing the participants. Two hours spent courting a potential mate will probably contribute more to your fu-ture happiness than twice that amount of time spent getting every last item out of your in-box after everyone else has gone home. And a yearlong commitment to one hour of community service at the same time each week is worth a great deal more to a nonprofit organiza-tion than a single donation made in cash representing your hourly wages for the same amount of time over the course of a year.

This is true not just because you're making it possible for that or-ganization to accomplish some unpopular task at below-market rates. (Don't make the mistake of thinking that your labor is free—the non-profit had to recruit you, after all, and coordinate your effort.) Nor is it true merely because it is worth something to a nonprofit to be able to make up a schedule in advance and stick to it. Your commitment adds value to that nonprofit, and to your town, and to your nation, be-cause, as you get to know a like-minded group of people and let them know that they can trust you, you form bonds with your neighbors and maybe even create a group where none existed before. You're adding to what economists call human capital and building what Third World development specialists call civil society.

4.
___

THE TORAH, otherwise known as the Five Books of Moses, tells the tale of God's efforts to fashion for himself a Chosen People. Moses' task is to extract a nation out of a rabble of former slaves. He has to create a civil society. In this mission, he fails. His failure, I believe, explains one of the great mysteries of the Bible: why God insists that Moses must die before his people enter the Promised Land.

What did Moses do wrong? When he asks God, God tells him that he struck a rock to make it yield water when he was supposed to speak to it—"because ye sanctified me not in the midst of the children of Israel." Millions of young Bible students have stopped reading at this point, appalled. One tiny infraction and Moses is denied entry into the Promised Land? Ask yourself, though: Why did he strike the rock? Because the people were thirsty, angry, and rebelling against him. Why were the people rebelling against him? Because they doubted God's ability to provide for them in the desert. Why did they keep doubting, when God had come through for them so many times? Because they were not yet a people who placed their trust in the Lord.

Another way to explain it is to say that Moses had not yet manufactured social cohesion. The Sabbath plays a small but important part in his effort to do so. In the book of Exodus, God gives the Israelites the Sabbath. The day makes its first appearance in their midst with a curious absence of fanfare. Its arrival is eclipsed by a more miraculous gift: manna, the breadlike substance that God deposits on the ground every morning, along with the dew, for the children of Israel to eat as they wander in the desert.

Six weeks out from Egypt, their provisions gone and nothing but sand as far as their eyes can see, the Israelites panic. They murmur, as the Bible puts it, against Moses and Aaron, exclaiming, "Would to God we had died by the hand of the Lord in the land of Egypt, when we sat by the flesh pots, and when we did eat bread to the full; for ye have brought us forth into the wilderness, to kill this whole assembly with hunger." God hears their complaints and tells Moses that he will "rain bread from heaven," and that the people should go out and gather only a certain amount every day.

Why not let everyone run out and grab as much as he can, and store it in case of need? God explains: He wants to test the people. He wants to see whether the Israelites can be taught to follow rules—to "walk in my law, or no." The law he has in mind is that of sharing, fairly, a scarce resource. So important is this lesson that God presses the manna into service as an instrument of pedagogy. The next morning, when the people go out to collect the stuff, each of them will come back with exactly one portion—one *omer*—no matter how much he plucked from the ground. That night, all uneaten manna will spoil, demonstrating the ill-advisedness of hoarding.

But God is not finished making demands. On the sixth day after the manna's first fall, he says, the people should gather twice as much as they do every other day. And that is all that God says by way of introduction to the Sabbath. His admonition goes by so fast that Moses doesn't even mention it to the people until the sixth day—an oversight so grave that the rabbinical commentator Rashi says it gave God another reason to punish him. But the idea of gathering twice as much on Friday sounds, at first, arbitrary, like an exercise in discipline rather than something worth doing on its own merits.

At this point, we have to turn back a few pages in the Book. Right before the miracle of manna takes place, another miracle occurs that is nearly identical to it. Three days after leaving Egypt, having found no water, the Israelites come across a spring that proves too bitter to drink, and murmur, in the Bible's verb, "against Moses, saying, What shall we drink?" Moses turns to the Lord, who shows him a tree that would, if thrown into the water, make it potable. Moses throws it, and they drink. Then and there, the Bible adds, God makes "for them a statute and an ordinance." Which statute and which ordinance? The Bible fails to say. The rabbis speculate that *that* was really the moment when God gave them the Sabbath. Maybe, maybe not, but the plain meaning of the passage is that God dreams up on the spot the very idea of the tit for tat. He imposes statutes and ordinances on the people in exchange for giving them the means of survival.

From God's breast issues the manna, which is as white as coriander seed and tastes like "wafers made with honey" and mysteriously manages to satisfy everyone's needs. ("What is it but heavenly, sweet, creamy milk that allows the entire congregation to nurse at once?" the commentator Ilana Pardes muses.) In return, God expects the self-restraint without which collective life would be impossible. As God gives to them, so they should give to him; and as God shares his bounty with them, so should they share it with one another, distributing it justly.

Of that lesson, the Sabbath can be said to be the perfect test, for it poses fundamental questions about social coexistence. Have the people grasped the principle of reciprocal altruism? Have they applied those principles with enough rigor and evenhandedness that individuals feel they can afford to stop competing for resources for an entire day? Are they comfortable enough with one another that each person doesn't feel he has to rush out and grab some manna before the next guy does?

The answer is no. "And it came to pass," the Bible goes on, "that there went out some of the people on the seventh day for to gather, and they found none." God, not yet used to being defied, fumes, "How long refuse ye to keep my commandments and my laws?" Then he states the rule again: "Abide ye every man in his place, let no man go out of his place on the seventh day." And so, the Bible says, "the people rested on the seventh day." But they obey God more out of fear than out of mutual trust.

This, by the way, is not the last we hear about the social dimensions of the Sabbath. Another cautionary tale appears in the book of Numbers, and it is even more disturbing. In it, God resorts to more punitive tactics. The Israelites come upon a man gathering wood on the Sabbath and bring him to Moses and Aaron, who don't know what to do with him. They take him into custody, and then they seek God's advice. He gives them a shocking answer: "The man shall be surely put to death: all the congregation shall stone him with stones without the camp."

Even the rabbis were taken aback by the severity of the sentence. In the Bible, religious violations often incur the ultimate penalty. But there are two kinds of ultimate penalty in the Bible, one executed by man and one by God; sins against man are almost always punishable by man, and sins against God are almost always punishable by God. The divine corollary to the death penalty, a punishment executed by human hands, is *karet,* or "cutting off." He who flouts God's law, according to the legal formula, will have his soul "cut off from among his people." The exact meaning of "being cut off" has been the subject of much debate: some have said childlessness; some an early death; some that the soul dies with the body, so that the culprit may not join his kin in the hereafter. What is clear is that the divine penalty differs from capital punishment, and it is left to God to execute it.

In a rare instance of double jeopardy, though, violations of Sabbath law incur both human and divine penalties. What makes God so harsh in his enforcement of the Sabbath? He must have considered violation of the Sabbath to be an offense against man as well as himself. A man gathering wood on the Sabbath is not only doing forbidden work; he violates the mutual non-compete clause that lets Sabbath-keepers feel they can afford not to work. If he gets away with it, then everyone else can, too, and no one will be able to rest. It will no longer be feasible to keep the Sabbath, and that, in the biblical construction of the holiday, indicates that no higher form of social order can be maintained.

5.

MODERN JERUSALEM IS A GOOD PLACE to go to think about the Sabbath's social efficacy. Jerusalem on a summer Saturday can stun you with its sweetness—its taste of the world to come, the rabbis liked to say—or leave you sweaty and bored. It depends on how you spend it. If you follow the flow of foot traffic to some gorgeous old synagogue packed with enthusiastic young Jews, then get yourself invited to a leisurely luncheon underneath a spreading tree, you may thank the God who invented the Sabbath and the rabbis who made it the law of the land. If you're stuck with two sick children in a guesthouse that serves no meals on Saturday, as I once was, you'll be less grateful.

Keeping the Israeli Sabbath is hard work, even if you aren't a tourist, particularly if you're unmoved by its pleasures. Hence the dislike of many secular Israelis for Saturday—the streets cleared of buses, the shuttered grocery stores and pharmacies, the understaffed hospitals—as well as for the black-hatted men in ultra-Orthodox neighborhoods who stone Sabbath-breakers and riot against the opening of parking lots, and who have in Israel's half century of existence twice nearly brought down governments that violated Sabbath laws. And hence my surprise when I learned that other secular Israelis have begun to treat the Sabbath as a national treasure in need of preservation.

In a column in *The Jerusalem Post* in 2002, the writer Hillel Halkin, who is not exactly religiously observant, noted that so many Israelis now shop at malls on Saturday that it seemed silly to complain about it—and then he complained about it. (Hundreds of stores at Israel's malls violate Saturday-closing laws, and Saturday has become the biggest shopping day of the week.) As a struggling writer and a father of two, Halkin said, he used to take solace from the ban on getting and spending, especially on Friday nights—the only night of the week that he failed to wake up in a panic "because the next day was a day on which you could not do anything about money anyway." A week without a break from acquisitiveness, he added, rather grandly, "is bad for the human spirit and it is bad for Israeli society."

Several prominent secular Israeli intellectuals have lately expressed the same thought. Like Halkin, and like American adherents to the volunteer simplicity movement, these secular Israeli Sabbatarians want to save the Sabbath from consumerism. They also want to remove it from the exclusive control of Israel's Orthodox rabbis. Ruth Gavison, a law professor at Hebrew University who has been working with a prominent Orthodox rabbi to draft a proposal for a less stringent Sabbath, told me that devising a Sabbath that even the non-pious could enjoy was part of a larger effort to rescue Israeli society. From what? I asked. From the widening chasm between secular and religious Israelis, and also from those who no longer see a rationale for a Jewish state, she explained. What does the Sabbath have to do with the legitimacy of Israel? I asked, somewhat surprised. A viable Jewish state must have an authentically Jewish public culture, she replied.

At the legal level, Gavison's idea is simple. She would codify permission for much of the non-commercial activity that already goes on and enforce the pause in commercial activity and industry already prescribed by law. Restaurants, concert halls, art galleries, and movie theaters would stay open—not just in cities and towns that have made special arrangements to do so but throughout the country. Buses would run, which they do not do now. Malls would be closed.

It is not as easy to understand Gavison's vision of a unifying Jewish public culture. She isn't sure herself what she means. Like many Israeli intellectuals, who model themselves on their European, not their American, counterparts, Gavison takes a high-minded approach to culture. She imagines bigger audiences for music, art, and theater; more meetings of affinity groups; more salons devoted to Jewish texts. One Jewish holiday celebrated in a semisecular way that might serve as an example is Shavuoth, which commemorates God's giving of the Torah to Moses at Sinai. It's an occasion marked by all-night study sessions held not just at synagogues but also at theaters and conference centers and other public venues. I once happened to be in Jerusalem for Shavuoth, and I saw the streets come alive at 11 P.M. with the rather astonishing apparition of Israelis of all kinds, not just the religious, roaming from lecture to lecture in small groups under the Jerusalem moon, seeking enlightenment on both the Bible and contemporary politics.

This, too, is an old vision of the Sabbath. The Sabbath, wrote the Babylonian scholar Saadia Gaon, "affords men leisure to meet each other at gatherings where they can confer about matters of their religion and make public pronouncements about them, and perform other functions of the same order." But Gavison's reference point is Ahad Ha'am, the late-nineteenth-century Zionist who argued for a cultural, rather than a political, Zionism—an Israel based on a positive Jewishness rather than on ethnic nationalism and anti-anti-Semitism. What he was calling for isn't clear, either, though anyone who has ever found himself on a synagogue mailing list will be familiar with his sociological aperçu: "More than Israel has kept the Sabbath, the Sabbath has kept Israel."

Can a day of rest really strengthen the bonds of a nation, or is that grandiloquence? Throughout the nineteenth and much of the twentieth century, Americans debated the merits of the Sabbath with the same passion that Israelis bring to it today, and on largely the same grounds. The discussion turned on the question of whether there was anything about Sunday that warranted preservation once the old Puritan rigor had lost its appeal. The secular answer was that the American Sunday had become indispensable to the task of fostering America's exceptional qualities—its egalitarianism and pluralism.

In a famous 1872 speech pleading for the opening of libraries and for public transportation on Sundays, the minister and abolitionist Henry Ward Beecher argued that only the liberalization of the Sabbath would conserve its character as a "a day peculiarly American" in its serendipitous neighborliness, family-minded "household love," moral uplift, and "poetic element." (Beecher was not above mixing xenophobia into his praise for the American Sunday. "Look at the countries where there is no Sunday," he said. "Yes, look at the countries where people are not educated. Look at the countries where the people are priest-ridden. Look at the countries where there is no popular liberty. There you find that the tyrant, whether he be hierarch or potentate, pays off the people for their political liberty by giving them holidays to play on. They please them with amusement on Sunday, and other bribes, to make them willing to part with their privileges. But that is not the case in this country.")

In 1906, an Episcopalian minister in Boston claimed, portentously, that Sunday had given the American character its "moral earnestness . . . that utters itself in every grand institution of freedom" and allowed "eighty million persons, the refugees of every land" to unite into a single people. In 1961, the Supreme Court justices Earl Warren and Felix Frankfurter issued separate but concurring opinions in defense of Sunday-closing (or blue) laws in a case called *McGowan et al. v. Maryland,* which wrote into legal history the bond between the Sabbath and civic consciousness. It's unsettling to remember how recently Americans couldn't work or shop on Sunday, except when medically necessary or when certain services or stores were deemed essential to fun on days off. What was wrong with letting people shop? Frankfurter glossed over the obvious point that it forced everyone in the retail sector to work and emphasized instead something less tangible: the bustling, humming feel of a street open for business, which, he said, had the power to destroy "a cultural asset of importance: a release from the daily grind, a preserve of mental peace, an opportunity for self-disposition." Warren and Frankfurter maintained that the Protestant Sunday had evolved into a secular day of recuperation, a public good that promoted the health of the American people and the orderliness of its society. Therefore, they ruled, blue laws did not violate the First Amendment's stricture against the establishment of religion.

6.

NEARLY FIFTY YEARS AFTER the Judahites were carried off to Babylon, Cyrus, the warrior king of the Persians, entered the city and took its puppet king prisoner. The Judahites hailed him as a savior. "He is my shepherd," Isaiah has God say of Cyrus. Cyrus sent the Judahites home to reestablish their government and rebuild their Temple. The Bible claims that Yahweh inspired Cyrus's generosity. Cyrus would have credited the principles of sound imperial administration. A shrewd and effective tyrant, he understood that he could ensure peace and stability in his kingdom by giving his subjects some control over their own destinies, but he handpicked their leaders to make sure that they were loyal to him.

The return took more than a century. The Judahites came in a trickle, then in waves. Their leaders were bookish, messianic, intense. Many of them hoped to restore the monarchy under Davidic rule. Rebuilding God's house did not just mean rebuilding his Temple and protecting it with walls. It also meant disentangling his people from the seductive embrace of non-Judahites. The efforts of these determined favorites of the Persian kings enraged the locals, many of whom had mixed happily with their polytheistic neighbors and even married some of them. The Judahites who had stayed behind had their own ideas of what it meant to be a Jew in a post-Temple world, and many of them harassed their new leaders. It should be noted that, right around this time, the returning Judahites begin to refer to themselves as "Jews," or "yehudin" in Aramaic—that is, residents of the colony the Persians called Yehud (Judah, in Persian).

Archaeologists disagree about exactly how many people really left Judah during the exile, how many remained, how many returned, and how returnees treated those who had been left behind. Most archaeologists doubt that the land ever lay as empty or ruined as the Bible makes it sound. But you don't need archaeology to see that, as a class, the "assembly of the exile" had little respect for the Jews who had remained in Yehud, and that these leaders devoted themselves to creating a special group of insiders free of all foreign influence and syncretism, and ensuring its dominance.

The Sabbath played a crucial role in this effort. The Sabbath was the great obsession of Nehemiah, a cupbearer and eunuch of the Persian king Artaxerxes sent to rebuild and govern Jerusalem in 445 B.C.E., and for Ezra, a priest and scribe sent by Artaxerxes to investigate the state of religious life in Yehud. (Ezra is the first person we know ever to stand up before a congregation—gathered, in this case, in front of Jerusalem's water gate—and read the Torah aloud.) Nehemiah and Ezra wanted to revive the cultic calendar, and started by enforcing Sabbath laws, which had largely been forgotten. "In those days," Nehemiah writes, "saw I in Judah some treading on wine presses on the sabbath, and bringing in sheaves and lading asses; as also wine, grapes, and figs, and all manner of burdens, which they brought into Jerusalem on the sabbath day. . . . There dwelt men of Tyre also therein which brought fish, and all manner of ware, and sold on the sabbath unto the children of Judah, and in Jerusalem." Horrified, Nehemiah complained to the city fathers, "What evil thing is this that ye do, and profane the sabbath day? Did not your fathers thus, and did not our God bring all this evil upon us, and upon this city?"

And so, Nehemiah tells us, he brought in his henchmen to block merchants from entering Jerusalem's gates. "And it came to pass, that when the gates of Jerusalem began to be dark before the sabbath, I commanded that the gates should be shut, and charged that they

should not be opened till after the sabbath: and some of my servants
set I at the gates, that there should be no burden brought in on the
sabbath day."

To understand how unneighborly it was for Nehemiah to shut
the city gates, you have to know something about the city gate in the
biblical world. It was much more than just a gate for going through or
keeping out. "It was also the 'center' (even though at one side) of the
city's social, economic, and judicial affairs," one historian writes. The
city gate and the street behind it functioned as the speaker's corner,
the town hall, the law court, and the marketplace, all at the same time.
That Nehemiah (or whoever wrote his book) understood the Sabbath as a way to winnow his people from the neighbors becomes clear
when you read the story immediately following it—in it, he yells at
the intermarried Jews and plucks their beards to prevent future inter-
marriage. After that dramatic illustration of his dislike of outsiders,
Nehemiah brings his story to a close. His second-to-last verse goes
like this: "Thus cleansed I them from all strangers."

7.

NEHEMIAH'S SHUTTING of the gates made the Sabbath a geographical
construct as well as a temporal one. The Sabbath, a day set apart, became a city enclosed, and a nation withdrawn into itself. Nearly a millennium later, the rabbis of the Talmud turned the Sabbath into a
more modern space, a place both enclosed and open. They developed
a body of laws whereby, by following certain prescribed procedures, a
community could construct a boundary marking off a Jewish neighborhood for the duration of the Sabbath. In lieu of a gate, the laws
called for a wall, but not the impermeable kind of wall that surrounded Jerusalem. This was not a wall of brick or clay or stone. This
was to be a notional wall—a wall concept, you might say, a boundary
marked by thin wires strung from pole to pole high above the head.
This wall-like entity they called an *eruv*, which in Hebrew means
"mixing" or "commingling," since an *eruv* brings together entities
otherwise kept apart on the Sabbath. (Technically, the word refers to

many acts that "mix" or "commingle" the forbidden with the permissible, not just this particular symbolic wall.)

The Bible wished upon its readers a very localized, confining Sabbath. Biblical law forbids Jews to walk very far or carry anything on the Sabbath from one domain to another. They are not to carry from the private domain, or home, to the public domain, or street, or the other way around, or between two private domains, and so on. The rabbinic *eruv* sweeps away these restrictions by bundling together assorted city spaces—apartment buildings and alleyways, courtyards and front yards—and recategorizing them, within limits, as one large private domain. (Busy public thoroughfares don't qualify.) The *eruv* advanced the legal fiction that all the Jews in a neighborhood live in one big *heimishe* Jewish household.

The potential for claustrophobic self-sequestration contained within this idea is, of course, enormous, and was often realized during the course of Jewish history, but its usefulness should also be pointed out. With an *eruv* in place, traditional Jews stroll through the streets on the Sabbath with a commanding ease, as if moving from room to room. Women carry their babies and push strollers; men carry their books and prayer shawls; guests carry wine to their hosts. At a more abstract level, an *eruv* delineates the contours of a Jewish space, which adds value beyond the value added when real-estate prices soar within the footprint of the *eruv*. If you read *Eruvin,* the tractate that deals with the laws of the *eruv,* you will discover that the rabbis belonged to, and wrote about, highly mixed societies. In their neighborhoods, Jews and non-Jews lived next to and on top of one another. Different kinds of Jews—rabbinic, non-rabbinic, Torah-reading, non-Torah-reading—also mingled. With the *eruv,* the rabbis uncovered a way to pry unity out of diversity. One set of *eruv* laws requires beneficiaries of an *eruv* to make a collective donation of bread, and imposes penalties on neighbors who are too stingy or forgetful to do so. As it was with collecting manna, so it is with building the *eruv:* You have to learn the lesson of cooperation. Another set of laws ponders the mystery of how to involve the non-Jewish neighbor in the peculiar act of making an *eruv.* The discussion concludes with the opinion that you

probably can't, and that you should probably retreat to a mostly Jewish neighborhood. The *eruv*, in other words, is a segregator and iden-
tity-enhancer and nation-builder. Its quasi-fictional walls were the
stage upon which the Jews imagined their way into the idea of community.

8.

SOMETIME IN THE MID-1970s, my mother, certain that our Puerto
Rican sojourn had weakened, if not destroyed, her children's sense of
Jewishness, began looking for a Jewish summer camp to send me to.
She wound up choosing the same summer camp that she had gone to
in the 1940s, an archetypal scattering of cabins, rec halls, and playing
fields in rural New Hampshire. This was the institution in which my
mother, a public-school student, had acquired her religious Zionism.
I did not appear likely to follow her example. I was a girl growing up
in the honky-tonk part of an American colony, used to spending my
spare time sneaking into hotels to swim in warm, clear, forbidden
pools. And suddenly I was forced to take swimming lessons in an ice-
cold dark-brown body of water that the instructors called a lake,
though it was clearly no more than a pond. My friends at home were
the transient children of businessmen briefly stationed on the island,
some American, some European. We had mastered the tone of world-
weariness meant to let people know that we were well traveled, if a bit
neglected. My fellow campers, on the other hand, were earnest students at Jewish day schools from the decorous middle-class suburbs of
Boston. I had to play games I'd never heard of, like tetherball, and pretend to know something about the TV shows that were constantly alluded to, even though Puerto Rican television, at least then, broadcast
only a handful of American programs, all a year or so late and dubbed
into Spanish.

I could fake acquaintance with American pop culture, but I
couldn't fake being Jewish. My after-school Hebrew school left me
with hardly any knowledge of the language, whereas my peers could
read the Bible in the original. Nor did I know what to do when we

gathered to pray first thing in the morning. I was particularly confused by one move, a series of steps ending in some bows that were required at the beginning and end of the standing silent prayer called the Amidah. I usually tried to imitate the person praying in front of me, which made everyone behind me snicker.

The camp had been founded in the 1940s, along with dozens of others like it and scores of Jewish schools, in response to rising anti-Semitism in Europe as well as in America. Once America entered World War II, echoes of the Nazi attack on Jews began to be audible at home. Charles Lindbergh, the pilot and hero and right-wing isolationist, blamed the Jews for pushing America into war; radio talk-show hosts such as Father Charles Coughlin claimed that the Jews started the war to profit from it. Zionism went from being the cause of a small clique of radical intellectuals to being hugely popular among American Jews. And Judaism as a religious practice, which had lost a great many adherents to the jazzy freedoms of secular Americanness, began to gather followers back unto itself. American Jews, the theologian and sociologist Mordecai Kaplan declared, were returning to Judaism "like prodigal sons."

Parents began to fret about teaching their children how to be Jews. Jewish schools were an obvious answer. Jewish summer camps were a non-obvious one. We can all imagine why a school would appeal to a parent who wants to teach her child some specific body of knowledge, or inculcate a particular set of values, but what made camps so attractive requires a little more teasing out.

It is no coincidence that in the 1940s experimental social psychology, whose practitioners invent dramatic and intense situations to study how groups affect individuals and vice versa, began to take an interest in camps. Nor should it be a surprise that American social psychology entered its heyday when refugees from Nazism began to arrive. The social experiment that was Nazism, the astounding transformation of ordinary Germans from enlightened-sounding democrats to regimented bystanders to mass murder, made it clear to everyone who had lived through it that there was such a thing as a group psyche, that it could turn individual psyches inside out, and that it could be manipulated. (And then, of course, there were those *other* camps.) Kurt Lewin, who did more than anyone else to convince psychologists that they ought to be studying the workings of power within and among groups rather than limiting themselves to individuals—he invented the term *group dynamics*—fled Germany in 1933, when Hitler came to power.

Muzafer Sherif was born in Turkey and studied at Harvard, but returned to teach in Turkey. Before he got there, though, he attended lectures at the University of Berlin, where Hitler was in his political ascendancy. Sherif wrote extensively about the dangers of Nazism, and when his books were published in Turkey, technically a neutral country for most of the war, he was thrown into jail. Influential friends from Harvard got him out, and by 1944 he was teaching at Yale.

Lewin's preoccupation was socialization—how individuals reconcile themselves to the mores of the group. His best-known study was of a boys' club, in which he showed how different styles of leadership—autocratic, democratic, laissez-faire—can reliably produce entirely different kinds of groups. Lewin saw that the value of camps for indoctrination lay in their isolation, in their being cultural islands, which allowed them to create alternate societies without interference from the dominant society. Isolation helped minimize resistance to new and different ideas.

Sherif was curious, among other things, about how groups develop norms; that is, values and standards of behavior, as well as a sense of who's in and who's out. He answered these questions by staging experiments in actual summer camps. In 1954, Sherif and his wife led one of the most famous experiments in social psychology, the Robbers' Cave experiment, named after the state park in Oklahoma that surrounded the two-hundred-acre Boy Scouts of America camp the Sherifs borrowed for their "summer camp." Anyone who has lived through a summer camp "color war" will recognize the Robbers' Cave experiment as an only slightly exaggerated version of the same thing. It involved two busloads of twelve-year-olds, all well-adjusted boys from similar backgrounds: lower middle class, white, Protestant.

Over the course of three weeks, the boys were made to form groups to which they became passionately attached, developing distinctive rituals and coming up with emblems, such as flags and ways of tying knots. Then they were incited to compete, which they did with ferocity and personal bitterness. And, in the end, they were led to make up. This last part took a long time and happened only after they were made to work toward common goals of great importance to all of them (restoring the camp's water supply, raising enough money to rent a movie).

The Sherifs may have intended to make a point about how we learn to love, hate, and get along, but they also provided robust evidence that the summer camp—a wholly controlled environment in which adolescents dwell far from parents, classmates, and the media for weeks, even months—is a remarkably efficient instrument of psychological manipulation. One of the most interesting features of the Robbers' Cave experiment has been pointed out by two contemporary social psychologists: The campers "perceived the environment as natural and had no awareness of the study or the staff's manipulations." The setting may have been artificial, but the participants experienced it as real; in social-psychological terms, it had high "experimental realism."

I have always wondered why summer camps aren't viewed with greater suspicion. Even plain-vanilla secular summer camps have their ideological agendas. As Abigail Van Slyck points out in her history of American summer camps, *A Manufactured Wilderness,* from the beginning camps were designed to fight back against the moral and physical degradations of city life. Camping has always been about counterprogramming to correct for some unsalutary influence.

Unlike the Sherifs' campers, I made my counterprogrammers work hard. I skulked around the bunk, complaining to anyone who would listen about being forced to participate. I was particularly scornful of the thrice-weekly Hebrew classes, where my ignorance was publicly exposed, and team sports, where I was every team's last pick. I was horrified when I learned that on Friday afternoons we marched down to the showers in our robes and towels and scrubbed ourselves especially clean, then dressed up in blouses and skirts for Friday-night dinner. This was regimentation of the most odious kind. Plus, the girls in my bunk fought one another for access to our few electrical outlets and comparatively scarce mirrors. They wanted to blow-dry their hair into just the right kind of flip and apply the modicum of makeup they were allowed to wear. Then they'd try on one another's skirts, swapping them in a round-robin so that they could appear to have new outfits each week, rather than just the one or two they'd brought from home. Hypocrisy! I thought. Didn't these Jews know that excessive self-regard is a sin?

As the weeks passed, I began to soften. I liked being clean once a week, and smelling everyone else's sharp clean smell. I looked forward to the meal, which featured challah and roast chicken and potatoes and cake, rather than the usual mess-hall stews and spaghetti, and was served on plates and tablecloths rather than on trays and bare tables. I got to know the songs and prayers well enough to bang on the table at the appropriate moments, even if I didn't have the nerve to look enthusiastic or sing. After dinner there was Israeli folk dancing, which was cheesy and dispelled the charm, though years later I still hum the tunes.

On Saturday mornings, though, there was no loudspeaker blasting Israeli pop songs to wake us up. We were relieved of the burden of a formal breakfast. In the afternoon, there were hours of respite from planned camp activities, time in which you couldn't do anything to win points against the other bunks. You couldn't clean up your bunk, or lengthen your lanyards, or work on your group's theatrical productions, or even acquire your fellow bunkers' savings by beating them at jacks, my one good sport. All you could do was alleviate your boredom. You lay around and chatted or, if no one wanted to talk to you, you wandered off for an hour or two by yourself to marvel that the sites of your daily striving—the waterfront, the softball fields, the study cabins—could seem so pastoral in the absence of counselors and whistles and scoreboards. The Sabbath of summer camp, because everyone around you observed it, too, felt much more real than any

Sabbath I'd ever experienced in the real world, where my mother and my siblings and I seemed to be the only ones who even noticed it.

Because I spent so much of it on my own, the Sabbath was also the only day of the week in which popularity and the lack thereof failed to dominate my consciousness, when I didn't have to pretend to be indifferent to status rankings whose minute calculations I apprehended in their utmost complexity. I could just *be* indifferent, at which point, of course, being indifferent no longer seemed so necessary.

So that was what I took away from camp at the end of the summer: the relief of my weekly respite from it. That, and something like a friend. My bunk's head counselor, Marjorie, who was headed to Brandeis that fall, began giving me books to carry off on my Saturday expeditions. These were mostly fairly standard college-freshman fare, which means there was a lot of Kurt Vonnegut. One Friday night, though, she handed me her copy of Karl Marx's *Communist Manifesto.*

This is not a story about how summer camp made me a Communist, because it didn't, although later, inevitably, as a teenager experiencing adolescent rage before the fall of the Soviet empire, I would fling Marxist-Leninist jargon at my father and conflate my own alienation with that of the proletariat. What *The Communist Manifesto* inspired was a fascination with the idea of the community that sets its face against the world and defines reality for itself. I picked this up from Marx's riff about "Critical-Utopian Socialism," which had something to do with people named Owen and Fourier. Actually, though this went over my head at the time, Marx was ranting against these men, ridiculing their utopian dreams as small-minded, counter-revolutionary, doomed to failure. To me, though, the nineteenth-century idylls he mocked sounded, well, idyllic, with names like "Home Colonies," "Little Icaria," "New Jerusalem." I was coming across this not long after the heyday of the hippie commune. I'd had no idea that the hippies hadn't been the first to come up with the idea. The utopias Marx described were like lively line drawings accompanying a dry, dull text. They made the revolution imaginable, and since I couldn't seem to be a member of the community I found myself in, I wanted to be a part of that one. These were the *real* summer camps, the Platonic ideals (not that I knew from Platonic ideals) of which my camp was but a wishful shadow. They were genuinely communal, genuinely remote, genuinely un-fallen from grace. In them, one might, on a permanent basis, achieve the kind of Sabbath my camp leaders were always talking about, one freed from the evil machinery of exploitation, rather than the corrupted, fashioncentric, Zionist Sabbath of actually existing Jews.

On the other hand, if you had to live among actually existing Jews, the New Hampshire summer-camp Sabbath seemed preferable to the August in Puerto Rico Sabbath. That fall and winter, I wrote my camp counselor friendly letters, telling her what I'd been reading, and in the spring, when my mother asked me if I wanted to go back the following summer, I said yes.

PART THREE

The Scandal of the Holy

1.

WHAT *IS* THE SABBATH, ANYWAY? YOU COULD CALL IT A *RELIGIOUS* institution—most people do—but its association with religion is in part an accident of history. The Sabbath is a relic of the days when most collective experiences were choreographed by professional clerics. You'd be safe if you called it a *social* institution, since society is a multiplication of the bonds that people weave among themselves, and the Sabbath helps tie such bonds, like a sort of sociological loom. You might characterize it as a *legal* entity, which is how the *yeshiva bocher,* the student of the Talmud, is taught to think of it. After all, for the Sabbath to exist at all there must be a set of rules that ensure that people don't work, and that those who don't work won't suffer for it. You might deem the Sabbath a *cultural* institution. If you wanted to make Sabbatarians of people who are fond of music and art, you would do well to explain to them that by setting aside one day in seven for non-employment they erect a temporary cultural venue for themselves, a concert hall in time. Or you could call the Sabbath a *political* institution. It makes the radically egalitarian claim that everyone—men, women, children, strangers, *and* animals—has the right not to work. The Sabbath asserts the fundamental dignity of the human being, beyond his or her productive function.

But the Sabbath has another definition. It's also a *holy* day. Thomas Shepard, a seventeenth-century American Puritan minister, is very emphatic about this: "The word *Sabbath* properly signifies not common but *sacred* or *holy* rest." God said it from the slopes of Mount Sinai: "Remember the sabbath day, to keep it holy."

If it strikes us as strange that this commandment comes before "Honor thy father and thy mother," that's not just because the Sabbath seems less germane to life today than does our relationship with our parents. It's because the words "keep it holy" no longer make sense to us. When people complain that they find praying to be an empty experience, that senselessness is what they're talking about. It's weird to fill your mouth with words that have been drained of meaning; it's like wrapping your tongue around a fossil. To those of us who live in a disenchanted, Euclidean world, the category of the holy feels like a superfluity, a drawer into which you might toss odds and ends. Sacred things are relics. Sacred words are abracadabra (the word is a parody of an Aramaic sentence describing God's act of creation: *avra ke'davra,* "I create as I speak"). Holy days, once meant to open up the heavens for a glimpse of time on a cosmic scale, are now "holidays," meant for skiing trips or preschool parties.

The notion that we're to keep the Sabbath holy—as opposed to just keeping it—makes it unpalatable to many Americans who might otherwise be eager to set aside one day a week for organized nonproductivity. Take Back Your Time, an American and Canadian group formed to push back against the encroachment of the work ethos, states its policy goals in the bureaucratese of the human resources professional, speaking of "time poverty relief" and "paid family leave" and "time for civic participation." This group and others like it, such as the volunteer simplicity movement, share a key objective—protecting people from the compulsion to overwork—with Sabbatarian organizations, such as the Seventh-Day Adventists, which fight to keep one day a week free using the constitutional tool of religious-accommodation law. Some of the non-religious groups also get funding and support from churches, synagogues, or religiously affiliated foundations. But they don't acknowledge it openly. The secular groups do not want the taint of the Fourth Commandment to scare unbelievers away.

Holiness scandalizes, as well it should. It's the very incarnation of unreason. Once Isaac Newton convinced us that time was a mathematical quantity, wholly measurable, infinitely divisible, and expressible in numbers, and economists showed us that time could be a commodity, exchangeable for money, we were bound to find implausible the notion that certain times were holy while others weren't. How could some points on a graph be charged with supernatural power while others rest inert? Where, precisely, would the holiness lurk? If it can't be measured, how do we know it exists? Then there's what I call the non-commutability of sacred occasions—the conviction that specific periods of time (such as the twenty-five hours or so of the Sabbath) are sacred in and of themselves, and that you can't substitute one day for another, making a Thursday, say, stand in for a Saturday. That seems like a childish lapse into concrete thinking.

And yet we never really free ourselves from concrete thinking. Human beings make qualitative distinctions among kinds of time; that is one of the things that make us human. Animals do, too, of course, or at least they recognize that one time is different from another time—there is feeding time, and there is mating time. But we, unlike them, are conscious of time *as time*. We wouldn't even conceive of time as such, as something that moved forward or backward or back and forth, if we didn't slice it up into alternating units—tick, *then* tock.

"What is the origin of that differentiation?" Durkheim asked. The religious calendar, he answered. Durkheim's radical insight into religion was that what it made sacred was collective experience; religion also gave a subjective account of that experience. Religion, he said, is "the eminently social thing." How did societies learn the very act of making distinctions? By segregating the holy from the unholy. "The sacred thing is *par excellence* that which the profane should not touch, and cannot touch with impunity." And how could the calendar be used to help in this effort? By establishing a temporal rhythm of rites, festivals, and public ceremonies, the calendar held the sacred apart from the mundane. "There is no religion," Durkheim wrote, "and, consequently, no society which has not known and practised this division of time into two distinct parts, alternating with one another."

An anthropologist named Edmund Leach came up with a clever twist on Durkheim's take on holy time: He called it the time of false noses. "All over the world men mark out their calendars by means of festivals," Leach observed. "We ourselves start each week with a Sunday and each year with a fancy dress party." Why do we do it? Why "wear top hats at funerals, and false noses on birthdays and New Year's Eve?" Leach held that our intermittent masquerades create the sensation of time moving in a steady forward march—not merely, he argued, by marking off regular intervals between festivities but also, paradoxically, by making time swing like a metronome. Festive time lets us toggle between social personae, between our regular selves and our dress-up selves. We put on suits for church or graduation or a wedding and become higher-status versions of ourselves. We don skeleton masks or superhero costumes for Halloween and enter the realm of death and the uncanny.

Holy time, then, is time that we ourselves make holy—time that we sanctify *by means of our selves.* We have to commit ourselves to holy time before it will oblige us by turning holy. How do we sanctify the Sabbath? By wearing a special robe, said the rabbis. By beautifying ourselves and our homes.

From this perspective, Sabbath rules can be seen as formal exercises in sanctification. Don't do on that day whatever it is that you do on all the other days. What could be less enchanting than that? By divvying up the world into *this* kind of activity and *that* kind of activity, we fabricate holiness. The atheist would say that this proves that religion is a charade. The rabbis would say that this is how we become like God. After all, God ushered his world into being by dividing one thing from another: light from darkness, the heavens from the earth, and so on. Much of Jewish law flows from the Durkheimian notion that drawing distinctions is a holy act. (It can't be irrelevant that

Durkheim, son and grandson of rabbis, spent some portion of his early education studying to be a rabbi.) On Saturday nights, for instance, once the sun has set and three stars have appeared in the sky, Jews mark the end of the Sabbath with a ritual called Separation (Havdalah), which involves lighting a braided candle and saying some blessings. One blessing reads, "Blessed are you, God, because you separate the holy from the everyday, the light from the darkness, the people of Israel from everyone else, and the seventh day from six days of creation."

2.

SAYING THAT HOLINESS PARTAKES of God is not to say that it is necessarily good. Contrary to what is implied in Sunday school, the biblical quality of holiness is not morally positive; it's morally neutral, rather like an electrical current. It can enliven or kill. God lets Moses glimpse him in the burning bush but does not reveal himself directly, for his unveiled presence could destroy the future liberator of the Jewish people. Holiness flows from one conductor to another. God gives his blessing to Abraham, who gives it to Isaac, who gives it to Jacob, who passes it on to his sons, who become the holy nation of Israel. This transmission is anything but a conventionally moral process. Abraham's and Isaac's wives Sarah and Rebecca, for instance, conspire against elder sons so that younger ones will receive their husbands' blessings—a clear violation of the rules of the society in which they live, and acts of deception that ought to bother us today. Sarah insists that Abraham leave Ishmael, his firstborn, and Ishmael's mother, Hagar, in the desert to die, in order to protect the inheritance of Sarah's son, Isaac. Rebecca tells her son Jacob to trick his father, the now elderly Isaac, into giving him a blessing rightfully owed to Esau, Jacob's ever-so-slightly older twin brother.

The matriarchs' behavior is indefensible, yet God defends it. He instructs Abraham to do as Sarah says, and after Jacob takes flight from an enraged Esau God comes to Jacob in a dream, blesses him, and tells him that he, too, like Abraham and Isaac before him, will father a great nation. The ethical strictures governing family and tribal life fade before the importance of choosing a person capable of carrying the blessing unto the next generation. "Divine election is an exacting and perhaps cruel destiny that often involves doing violence to the most intimate biological bonds," the critic Robert Alter writes.

Holiness, in the Bible, is not only family-unfriendly; it is socially discriminatory. Anyone who has ever studied the book of Leviticus, for example, has been stunned by the radical non-inclusiveness of its laws, which force lepers out of the community and make menstruating women taboo. "Holiness means keeping distinct the categories of creation," the anthropologist Mary Douglas writes. "It therefore involves correct definition, discrimination, and order." Animals with blemishes may not serve as sacrifices. The blind and the lame may not be priests. Women who have given birth and men who have ejaculated must purify themselves, because bodies that leak aren't whole.

You can construct a dark and alienated existentialism on the scaffolding of *qadosh,* with its implication of God's separating himself from us. The biblical scholar David Damrosch says that the Law, which creates "a principle of separation" between humans and animals, Jews and non-Jews, should be seen as "a metaphor for the transcendental otherness of God." But another way to think about that is to say that the laws of holiness make you continually aware that God lives in heaven and you don't.

3.
___

So how does the Bible explain the holiness of the Sabbath? It refers us to the story of Creation.

It is possible to summarize the Creation story as a set of answers to some basic questions. *Why is there something rather than nothing?* Because in the beginning God created. *Why is there what there is and not something else?* Because he created heavens, earth, sea, land, stars, moon, sun, plants, animals, and humans. *And why do we have the Sabbath?* Because when God was done creating he rested.

At this point, though, we circle back on ourselves. *Why did God rest?* Because he wanted to create the Sabbath. We still don't know why the Sabbath should be a part of Creation. To understand that, you have to know about P. P and J are the authors said by modern biblical scholars to have written the two accounts of Creation that open the book of Genesis. P wrote the version that starts at the beginning, with God creating the heavens and the earth, and J wrote the one that starts with the Garden of Eden and features Adam and Eve. P, who was also the law- and purity-obsessed author of the book of Leviticus, is thought to have been a priest living sometime in the fifth or fourth century B.C.E. Some scholars feel that P was not just P; he was also R, the Redactor responsible for stitching together the Five Books of Moses as we know them. A handful of scholars go further and claim that Ezra, the priest who first read the Bible as we know it to the assembled people of Israel upon his return from Babylon, was both P and R.

Whoever he was, P does not benefit by the comparison to J, whose supple story of Creation features Adam, Eve, the snake, and God circling around a tree in a dance of good and evil. P, by contrast, writes like a cleric. His prose reads less like a story and more like a sermon. He has no characters; he never descends to the human level. He perches with his God above the cosmos, laconic, untouchable.

One thing we can say in P's defense, though, is that he was Judaism's first philosopher. Call him the Jewish Aristotle. His account of Creation lacks J's subtlety but achieves the grandeur of keen analytical thinking. It begins as simply as a folktale and ends with the magnificence of church-organ Bach. Along the way, it offers a tantalizing glimpse of ancient science. P doesn't just tie the material world to the creativity of his First Cause; he categorizes God's creations. There are sea and sky and land; fish and birds and animals; beasts that run wild, beasts that can be domesticated, and beasts that crawl; and, of course, humans. P doesn't limit himself to the physical, either. His God creates the temporal, too, though he doesn't so much call forth the units of time as divide them one from the other. Light he creates, but then he divides day from night, allotting much light to day and a lesser amount to night. Evening is winnowed from morning. There is one day, then two days, then three, then six.

The most remarkable feature of P's protoscientific narrative, though, is that it leads us with every weapon at the poet's disposal—rhythm, repetition, parallelism—toward its conclusion: the seventh and final day. This is no accident. P is working out the details of a monotheistic cosmos, and the Sabbath would seem to be an essential element of it. Behold creation in all its magnificence, P appears to be saying. This can't be the work of some squabbling, inconsistent, all-too-human gods. It can only be the work of the one God who dwells beyond time and space, light and matter. The Sabbath is that dwelling.

To grasp where the Sabbath ranks in P's world, you have to compare the creation of things to the creation of time. As God creates things, he moves from the lowest (the creatures of the sea) to the highest (humans, made in God's image). As he ekes out the units of time, he also ascends. Each day has more acts of creation than the previous one, and each is deemed to be good, but still, the stakes get higher each time. On day six God creates man and woman, and that, he says, observing his handiwork with satisfaction, is "very good." At long last, we get to day seven. We reach the end of the week.

Whereupon God rests. It seems an odd thing to do. As endings go, it's pretty muffled. One way to interpret it is as a loud silence, a deliberate not-saying of something. That's how students of comparative religion explain the story. God's apparent passivity at the very peak of narrative excitement, they say, is covert commentary on a competing epic, the Enuma Elish, the Babylonian myth of Creation. In that saga, after the gods create men, they free themselves for leisure by creating men, turning them into slaves, and putting them to work. Then the gods celebrate. They throw a party. If you were making a Hollywood version of the Enuma Elish, you'd base the party scene on Fellini's *Satyricon;* you'd want that Roman orgy feel, with naked servants glueing their eyes to the ground. The God of the Bible, on the other hand, also rests after creating humans, but he doesn't turn them into slaves. On the contrary, when God gathers his people at Sinai and commands them to rest because he did, too, he will generously share with humanity what theologians call the "divine otiosas," the godly rest.

Another way to solve the riddle of the ending is to stay inside the biblical text, rather than search for answers outside it. At the end of Exodus, in a passage also ascribed to P, we find the language used to describe Creation—the same words, in more or less the same order—being used to narrate the construction of God's Tabernacle in the desert. Moses *sees* (same word) the *work* (same word) the people *did* (same word), and *blesses it* (just as God blessed man and woman when they were created). A rabbinic midrash, or imaginative meditation, puts it this way:

> The Tabernacle is compared to the whole world, which is called a "tent," just as the Tabernacle is called a "tent." How so? It is written, "In the beginning God *made*" and "He spreads forth the heavens like a *curtain*"; regarding the Tabernacle it is written, "And you shall *make curtains* of goatskin for the tent of the Tabernacle." Regarding the second day of Creation, it is written, "Let there be an expanse . . . that it may *separate* . . ."; regarding the Tabernacle it is written, "So that the curtain shall be for you a *separation.*" Regarding the third day, "Let the water beneath the heavens be gathered"; and regarding the Tabernacle, "Make a laver of copper and a stand of copper for it, for washing." Regarding the fourth day, "Let there be lights in the expanse of the sky"; and regarding the Tabernacle, "You shall make a lamp of pure gold." Regarding the fifth day, "and birds that fly above the earth"; and regarding the Tabernacle, "The cherubim shall have their wings spread." On the sixth day man was created; and regarding the Tabernacle, it is written, "You shall bring forward your brother Aaron." Regarding the seventh day it is written, "The heaven and the earth were *completed*"; and regarding the Tabernacle, "Thus was *completed* all the work of the Tabernacle." . . . Regarding the seventh day it is written, "God *completed*"; and regarding the Tabernacle, "On the day that Moses *completed.*" Regarding the seventh day it is written, "And he *sanctified* it"; and regarding the Tabernacle, "And he *sanctified* it."

When you imagine P writing about the Tabernacle in the desert, it's hard to conceive that he would not have been thinking about the

Temple in Jerusalem. Ancient Israel, in its priestly days, was a Temple society, organized socially, economically, and theologically as a series of concentric circles radiating outward from the holy of holies in the middle of the Temple sanctuary—an empty, silent space that no one but the high priest had leave to enter, and he only once a year. When P had God withdrawing to the Sabbath, he must have imagined God entering this most sacred of all spaces.

Which makes the ending suitably grand. God enters his palace and ascends his throne. The medieval Jewish liturgists adored this image; they called the Sabbath God's coronation. The ancient rabbis dwelled just as lovingly on the echoes between the Temple and the Sabbath, though they expressed their critical insight in a typically oblique fashion. They said that the thirty-nine main categories of work forbidden on the Sabbath—known as *melachah*—derived from the thirty-nine kinds of work done to build the Tabernacle in the desert, labor that was also called *melachah*.

Ironically, the thirty-nine categories of *melachah* don't have much to do with the kinds of work needed to build God a home in the desert. It's likely that the prohibitions evolved over centuries as a kind of rough compilation of categories of work performed in everyday life in an agricultural society. (The thirty-nine categories are plowing, sowing, reaping, binding sheaves, threshing, winnowing, selecting or sorting, sifting, grinding, kneading, cooking, shearing animals, washing or bleaching or wringing a wet garment, carding, dyeing, spinning, chainstitching, setting up the warp or drawing it through the heddles, weaving of any kind, unravelling, tying a knot, untying a knot, sewing, ripping, catching game, slaughtering, flaying an animal, tanning, scraping the skin or smoothing, marking it up, cutting, writing, erasing, building, demolishing, kindling, extinguishing, beating with a hammer, which is interpreted as striking the last blow or applying the finishing touch to something, and carrying from the public to the private domain, or vice versa.) Only retrospectively would these categories of work have been applied to the Tabernacle by the rabbis.

Nonetheless, the association between *melachah* and Tabernacle makes poetic sense. By stopping work on the Tabernacle, we imitate God when he stopped working on the world. We, too, enter into the Temple. This image allows the rabbis, in the centuries after the Romans burned and looted the Jewish people's most sacred space, to erect the Sabbath in its place. It is another of the ironies of the rabbinic Sabbath that it replaced a structure with a holy hole in its middle, for the holiness of the Sabbath lies in its being a not-doing in a not-place.

4.

But the Bible has not finished telling us about the holiness of the Sabbath. There is a hole in the hole, a mystery inside the mystery, a holy of holies.

You'd think that, by the end of the story of Creation, we would be done. God made the universe in six days and took his place at its center on the seventh. If ever there were an image of plenitude, this would be it. Time and space have been spun into separate webs and brought back together in a seamless totality. God has exercised his creative power to its fullest. And yet, at this very moment, the story takes a twist. There is apparently one more thing for God to do. God does not stop working entirely on the seventh day. *First* he finishes the work that he has been doing. *Then* he stops doing the work that he has been doing (the Bible's repetition, not mine) in order to bless and sanctify the seventh day.

"His work!" the rabbis cried in alarm. What work? Didn't God finish Creation on the sixth day? What remained for him to finish on the seventh? How can P, that inveterate divider, that adamant classifier, allow work to run over from the mundane days to the holy one, contaminating and confusing the categories of sacred and profane, rest and work?

In the midrash that raises this question, the rabbis phrase their question rabbinically, which is to say, as a matter of legal concern: How could God have violated his own Sabbath by completing his work on that day? Rabbi Ishmael ben Jose declares, "It is like a man striking the hammer on the anvil, raising it by day and bringing it down by nightfall"—that is, after the start of the Sabbath, at which point, according to the rabbis, you may not put the finishing stroke on a piece of work (the thirty-eighth *melachah*) even if that means you have to stand there for twenty-five hours with your arm sticking up. Rabbi Simon ben Yochai shrugs the contradiction away. God's ways are God's ways, he says. Man can't be expected to have as keen a sense of time as God and has to stop work early to avoid violating the Sabbath. But God gets to enter the Sabbath by a hairbreadth if he wants to.

A rabbi named Genibah offers a more satisfying explanation. The verb "finish" and the noun "work," he says, are there to teach us that Sabbath rest is not just a nothing, a not-doing, but a something that requires creating. "This may be compared," Genibah continues, "to a king who made a bridal chamber, which he plastered, painted, and adorned. Now what did the bridal chamber lack? A bride to enter it. Similarly, what did the world lack? The Sabbath." Another rabbinical aphorism: God's creating the world is like a king who made a ring. What did it lack? A signet, or, one might say, a signature. (There is a shrewd truth to his insight: Creation myths in every other religion also account for the earth, the sky, plants, animals, and humans, but only the Jewish God created the Sabbath. It's his signature.) What unique entity was created through God's act of rest? Rest itself: "tranquility, ease, peace, and quiet."

Nonetheless, the rabbis don't solve the mystery of what, precisely, God is up to on the seventh day. They can't. It's an opacity in an otherwise transparent story. God turns his back on us and occupies himself with something that's even more important to him than we are. We are not privy to the details.

To understand the implications of God's choosing to absorb himself in the otherness of the Sabbath, we have to turn to the second story of Creation, which comes next. You know how it goes. God forms Adam out of dust, breathes into his nostrils, plants a garden for him, puts the tree of knowledge of good and evil right in the middle, and forbids man to eat from it. Afraid that Adam might get lonely,

God makes the animals. When that fails to yield companionship, he takes Adam's rib and fashions woman. Adam and Eve live together in perfect happiness, naked and unashamed, until the moment, which one imagines occurring on a long, lazy, slightly boring afternoon, with a primordially brilliant sun dancing on the leaves of the tree and the river that goes out from Eden gulping musically over the rocks, when the snake sidles up to Eve and asks, So you don't get to eat any of the fruit on these trees?

Eve shakes her head to correct him and says, "We may eat of the fruit of the trees of the garden. But of the fruit of the tree which is in the midst of the garden, God hath said, 'Ye shall not eat of it, neither shall ye touch it, lest ye die.' " That last bit—about God saying not to touch it—isn't true, but so eager to be informative is Eve that she embellishes the facts of the case.

Before you know it, Eve and Adam have eaten the fruit, realized that they were naked, flushed with embarrassment, and sewed themselves clothes out of fig leaves that look a lot like aprons. At which point God can be heard walking in the garden. It must be evening by now, because he is walking "in the cool of the day." Adam and Eve hide. God calls out to Adam, "Where art thou?"

Adam stutters, with the stupidity of a man caught red-handed, that's he's hiding because he doesn't want to be caught naked.

God asks, "Who told thee that thou wast naked? Hast thou eaten of the tree, whereof I commanded thee that thou shouldest not eat?"

Adam blames Eve.

God asks Eve, "What is this that thou has done?"

Eve blames the snake.

It doesn't occur to her to ask the question that seems obvious today: Where were *you,* God, that you need to ask such questions? Where were you when we innocents stumbled, as innocents will?

The usual explanation for God's apparently having been absent during Adam and Eve's fall from grace is that he wasn't. He asks Adam his whereabouts, but "the question is rhetorical," the philologist E. A. Speiser says in the Anchor Bible. Rashi works even harder to clear God's name. "God knew where Adam was!" Rashi declares. God asked Adam the question "only to engage in conversation with him, so that he not be too bewildered to repent."

The assumption behind Speiser's and Rashi's assertions is that God is omniscient and omnipotent, all-seeing and all-knowing. In forbidding Adam and Eve to eat from the tree, God gave humankind free will, for he gave them the means to transgress against him. They chose to transgress. Now, according to the theologians, God must play his parental role. He punishes Adam and Eve by expelling them from Eden, thereby teaching them right from wrong. But what if we declined to read theologically and simply read for plain sense? What if God weren't just pretending not to know for instructional purposes? What if he really didn't know? Then we'd have to ask, Where *had* he been all this time?

That is where P comes back in, at least insofar as he is also R, the Redactor. For in putting the two stories of Creation next to each other, by encouraging us to read the second as a fleshing out of the first—Creation as seen from a human perspective—P suggests an answer: God withdrew to take a nap. It is, after all, some time after the creation of man, which, by one accounting, might make it the seventh day.

I should note that the rabbis don't entertain such a blasphemous sequence of events. According to their reconciliation of the two stories, Adam and Eve were created and expelled on the same day: "They had enjoyed the splendors of creation but a brief span of time—but a few hours," as the midrash compiler Louis Ginzberg puts it. In the first hour of the sixth day, God conceived the idea of creating man. In the second hour, he took counsel with the angels. In the third, he gathered the dust for the body of man. In the fourth, he formed Adam. In the fifth, he clothed him with skin. In the sixth, the soulless shape was complete, so that it could stand upright. In the seventh, a soul was breathed into it; in the eighth, man was led into Paradise. And so on until the twelfth hour, when he was cast out of Paradise. The flaw in this reckoning, though, is that it doesn't give Adam time to fall asleep so that God can remove his rib and make Eve—indeed, it doesn't account for Eve at all. So in my midrash I say that it is the day of God's Sabbath, and he's having a *shabbas shluf*—a "Sabbath sleep." While he does that, the snake emerges. The air in the garden grows chilly. The story unfolds.

Whether the expulsion came before or after the first Sabbath, it was not a joyous day. It was, for Adam and Eve, God the Father's first show of indifference. Remembering the Sabbath and keeping it holy, for God, means abandoning his children to their own impulses. God's rest is man's fall.

5.

CAN WE DEFEND SABBATH HOLINESS by saying that it has social utility? The ancient rabbis would have disliked the question, since they didn't see the world in utilitarian terms, and they also didn't engage in open apologetics. But modern rabbis have been willing to be more explicit. Rabbi Samson Raphael Hirsch, the founder, in mid-nineteenth-century Germany, of what we now call Orthodox Judaism, glossed the Sabbath as a proto-environmentalist institution: "What was there to safeguard the world against man?" The answer is the Sabbath, because it checks his will to master the world. Man "can fashion all things in his environment to his purpose—the earth for his habitation and source of sustenance; plant and animal for food and clothing. He can transform everything into an instrument of human service," Hirsch wrote. "He is allowed to rule over the world for six days with God's will. On the seventh day, however, he is forbidden by divine behest to fashion anything for his own purpose. In this way he acknowledges that he has no rights of ownership or authority over the world."

The timing of this cautionary thought is suggestive. Hirsch wrote it down three decades before Karl Marx published *Das Kapital*. Both men lived at the height of the industrial age, when many feared the tyranny of automation and production schedules—the ideology called "productivism." What *melachah* ("mindful work") prohibited, said Hirsch, was purposiveness. It is a curious feature of the rules about *melachah* that they do not enjoin tasks that most of us would call work, or they offer loopholes that seem to circumvent their spirit. You

can throw a BarcaLounger across a room if you've got the muscles to
do it. You may do all kinds of things that are otherwise forbidden,
such as opening a carton of milk, if you do them in an apparently
counterproductive manner, such as cutting off the top of the milk carton so you can't close it again. If *melachah* requires "the execution of
an intelligent purpose," then it isn't just physical exertion, since you
can strain yourself silly without intending anything intelligent or purposive by your effort.

Likewise, you can't call an act *melachah* if it is done unconsciously
or unintentionally. Since *melachah* has to *make* something, destructive
acts don't count as *melachah,* either. The rabbis saw as clearly as
Durkheim did that it is people who create the distinction between
the holy and the unholy. *Melachah* is an act of mind as well as the work
of the body. There is no such thing as an intrinsically prohibited form
of Sabbath work. Every act is categorized according to the intention
behind it. If something is torn down so that something else can be
built in its place, that's *melachah,* but if it is torn down out of sheer de-
structiveness, it's not. If a woman puts out a fire to save a bit of wood,
that's *melachah,* but if she just wanted to put out the fire it's not. You
may not pluck flowers that you might put into water, or harvest
grindable grains of wheat, but feel free to pull dandelions or random
leaves of grass out of the ground and toss them aside, as long as you do
so thoughtlessly. (It should be noted that the rabbis qualify each of
these principles with countless exceptions, prohibiting many acts that
they might otherwise have permitted, on the theory that committing
these acts might *lead* to transgression. For instance, you should be able
to put out a fire as long as you don't mean to derive any positive benefit from doing so. However, the rabbis state that you must not extin-
guish a fire at all.)

You refrain from *melachah* to free your mind from the mental
work of getting things done. Now, Judaism is not a religion that dis-
dains getting things done. Judaism delights in both the pleasures of the
body (the five senses, sex, and drink) and the pleasures of the world
(clothes and homes and convivial conversation). From the sixth day of
Creation, humans have had orders in hand to be fruitful and multiply.

To do that, they had to enter enthusiastically into the world, not flee from it. Moreover, the Creation story makes no meaningful distinction between the artificial and the natural worlds, between civilization and biology. Humans were told to use the materials God gave them—the plants and the animals—to make themselves a home. By which we understand not just a house but a context, a culture, a way of constructing buildings and wearing clothes and cooking feasts and telling stories and making music and generally making something out of life.

So why stop building the world one day out of seven? The rabbis' answer—at least as Hirsch interpreted it—is, so that we don't forget that we, too, are creatures of God, and start imagining ourselves as masters of Creation. That resort to the deity, however, shouldn't impress us, since it doesn't explain *why* we're not supposed to see ourselves that way. What about *imitatio Dei*? What kind of God objects to competition from his creations? Shouldn't a father long for his children to outstrip him?

To come up with an answer less foreign to the secular mind, it helps to make use of categories dreamed up by a secular philosopher—by, as it happens, a secular German Jew, writing more than a century after Hirsch. In her masterwork, *The Human Condition,* Hannah Arendt offers another way of thinking about the rules against work on the Sabbath, although, being a determinedly godless Jew, she wasn't thinking about the Sabbath when she did. Arendt's aim was to explain what it means to be human. To that end, she posits the three "fundamental human activities": labor, work, and action. These, she says, "correspond to the basic conditions under which life on earth has been given to man."

Labor, says Arendt, is the struggle to subsist. It responds to the demands of biological life. "Labor assures not only individual survival, but the life of the species," she wrote. Tethered as it is to need, labor feels like enslavement, and indeed, throughout history, has been done by those who had no choice in the matter—slaves, women, the economically deprived. "Work" involves making things—tables, buildings, operas—that outlast the cyclical rhythms of labor. Work entails intention, design, and craftsmanship. Unlike labor, which is never done, work has a beginning and an end. Work, said Arendt, endures. It bestows "permanence and durability upon the futility of mortal life and the fleeting character of human time." Arendt's third activity, "action," is the vaguest of her categories. It seems to involve the public domain—speaking, legislating, governing, and founding and preserving political institutions. Arendt rated action the highest of the three activities, because it brings to the fore our uniquely human qualities. It uncovers in us potential we didn't even know we had. In so doing it "creates," she said, "the condition for remembrance, that is, for history."

Arendt's definition of *action* may have been fuzzy, but her bisection of *labor* and *work* was inspired. She came up with the idea, one suspects, to counter the influence of Marxism, since Marx glorified labor as the source of all value. Arendt felt that neither labor nor work deserved such honor. (Strictly speaking, Marx meant economic, not social, value, but Arendt is not wrong to imply that in reality Marxists esteemed labor and laborers above just about everything else.) Laboring, we restrict ourselves to our animal state. Working, we reduce the world to raw material. And if we take the work experience as the model for life itself, as economically minded thinkers have done since the advent of the industrial age, then we start to calculate all creation in terms of usefulness. *Homo faber*—Arendt's term for man the fabricator—thinks, she says, in terms of ends and means, of "in order to" rather than "for the sake of." In this way, he deprives himself of the capacity to see things as they are, for the sake of themselves.

But why should we *need* to see things as they are? And haven't we learned by now that it's impossible? But Arendt wasn't just talking about objectivity, which she defined philosophically as the thingness of things. She was talking about the ability to perceive in ourselves our human condition—the fact that we were born into this world and are destined to die. The human condition is the experience of *being conditioned* by the world. Our lives take their shape by virtue of being a part of the earth and all that abides in it—the earth being, according to Arendt, "the very quintessence of the human condition." And yet the earth is what humanity seems most eager to escape,

whether by rocket ship or the Internet. Having built the world by subjecting it to his will, *homo faber* now stands at risk of making it disappear. One of these days, his mastery of all will mean that he is confronted by nothing. And that will be a lonely day indeed.

The rabbis would not have approved of Arendt's mid-twentieth-century existentialist angst, nor would they have shared her Greco-Roman fetish for the agora, the marketplace of ideas or *action*. But their understanding of *melachah* dovetails with her definition of work. You might even say that the Sabbath laws were designed to show Jews that they were creatures of the earth, embedded in the time and place in which they were put by God (the rabbis' term) or the accident of birth (Arendt's term). Follow the rules and you'll see how well they produce this insight. Every other day of the week, you can extend your reach and enhance your control until you might as well be a cyborg—half man, half machine. On the Sabbath, the proscription of *melachah* strips you of those powers. You must respect the luminosity and aurality and architecture of the world that has been given.

6.

IF ALL THIS tempts you to develop a glorified view of the Sabbath, however, you need only read more history to remember that Sabbath holiness can be destructive as well as life-affirming. You can read about how the Sabbath became the object of a suicide cult.

Any American with a multicultural upbringing will recognize the outlines of the story, told every year at Hanukkah. In 167 B.C.E., Antiochus IV, a Syrian-born but Greek-educated king whose empire included Judea, decided to force the Jews to become more like the Greeks. This king called himself Antiochus Epiphanes (Antiochus the Manifest, meaning that he represented a divine emanation), but he was known to the people as Antiochus Epimanes (Antiochus the Mad). He was the first to introduce religious persecution to the region. Previous rulers had treated their subjects as sources of tax revenue; they had used force to extract their tributes, but they had not required conversion. Antiochus IV, however, had lived in Rome, and had seen Rome impose the Roman civic religion on its citizens. He had watched the Roman senators quash the local Dionysian bacchanalian cults, with their drunkenness and their fertility rites, and persecute the Epicurian philosophers, who preached a hedonistic doctrine that filled the young with subversive ideas. Antiochus regarded Judaism as an unholy combination of both cult and philosophy. Like members of a cult, Jews met at night, took loyalty oaths (the Shema, which pledged allegiance to the one God), and initiated new members through circumcision; like philosophers, they taught repugnant ideas out of books.

And so, the two books of Maccabees recount, Antiochus decided to "Hellenize" the Jews. He looted the Temple and garrisoned soldiers in Jerusalem. He put an idolatrous statue in the Temple (no one knows what it was; the books describe it only as "an abomination of desolation"), erected his own altars, and ordered the Jews to start sacrificing pigs on them. He forbade them to circumcise their sons or keep the Sabbath. "And whosoever would not do according to the commandment of the king," First Maccabees relates, "he should die." Women who had their babies circumcised in secret were killed, and the babies were hung from their necks. Their husbands were killed as well, and so were the men who performed the circumcisions. Anyone who refused to eat non-kosher food was killed.

Many of Jerusalem's urbane, partially Hellenized Jews did as Antiochus ordered, but the Jews of the countryside did not. Instead, they rebelled. Their leader was a priest named Mattathias, in a village called Modein. First Mattathias ran a spear through a Jew who agreed to sacrifice a pig on one of Antiochus's altars, then he said, "Whoever is zealous of the law, and maintaineth the covenant, let him follow me!" Mattathias had many sons, and they followed him into the desert. One of them was named Judah Maccabeus, and the rebels became known as the Maccabees. They took to the mountains and, improbably, drove the king and his soldiers out of the land.

Before that moment, however, retold every Hanukkah, came another that is decidedly not celebrated today. A large band of soldiers came down from Jerusalem to where a group of Jews identified only as the Pious Ones had shut themselves up in caves. (The word for Pious Ones is *Asidoi,* which is Greek for *Hasidim.*) When the Sabbath came, the soldiers lined up in front of the caves in battle formation and shouted, "Come forth, and do according to the commandment of the king, and ye shall live!" The Asidoi shouted back, "We will not come forth, neither will we do the king's commandment, to profane the Sabbath day!"

When the soldiers advanced, the Jews made no effort to block the entrances to the caves. Instead, they said to one another, "Let us all die in our innocence: heaven and earth shall testify for us, that ye put us to death wrongfully." The tale ends like this: "So they rose up against them in battle on the Sabbath, and they slew them, with their wives and children, and their cattle, to the number of a thousand people."

When Mattathias learned of the massacre, he quickly changed the laws of the Sabbath to permit self-defense, a rule that stands today, even in the strictest Jewish circles. The rule is called *pikuach nefesh,* or "saving a life." The Sabbath laws *must* be flouted if keeping them puts a life or the well-being of the community in danger—a principle that, for instance, allowed Senator Joseph Lieberman, a Sabbath-observant Orthodox Jew, to run for president of the United States. As he pointed out, he would have no qualms about violating Sabbath restrictions to respond to an attack or anything else that threatened the nation.

The story of the Maccabees and *pikuach nefesh* is sometimes told to show that the Jews understood full well that, as Christ put it, "the Sabbath was made for man, not man for the Sabbath." The truth, however, is that the Maccabees' reform was controversial at the time and remained unpopular for centuries. Some Pietists were so furious at Mattathias that they refused to fight for Judea's independence and went on to oppose his sons' rule, which lasted for eighty years and became known as the Hasmonean dynasty. The second book of Maccabees, for instance, written decades after the first book by someone who was clearly hostile to the Hasmoneans, offers a version of the war that leaves Mattathias out, as well as his modification of Sabbath law. The second book makes the Asidoi's Sabbath martyrdom seem laudable rather than tragic, for it offers a way to atone for Israel's sins, thereby hastening its redemption.

Indeed, the second book of Maccabees wallows in martyrdom. It speaks admiringly of women who, having circumcised their sons in violation of the law, are made to march around the city while nursing their children and are then forced to throw them over the city walls. The book tells the tale of a mother who urges her sons to refuse to eat pork. The king, enraged, mutilates them one by one. First their tongues and extremities are cut off; then they're burned alive. The mother exhorts each of them in turn, "Regard not your selves for God's sake." You understand people best by the literature they write, and in the second book of Maccabees the Jews invented a genre that would come to dominate Jewish, then Christian, literature: the martyrology.

You were supposed to die for the Sabbath, even if people rarely did. The Jewish historian Josephus praised Jews who sacrificed themselves to preserve the principles of the day, even though he later saved his own skin by decamping to the enemy during Rome's war against Palestine. Josephus was aware of the Maccabean revision of the law, but he chose to revert to the older version. The Maccabees had been willing to ambush their enemies on the Sabbath, taking advantage of their mistaken belief that Jews wouldn't fight. Josephus held that while Jews may respond to an attack on the Sabbath, they may not start one. Dying for the holiday may seem ridiculous to the uninitiated, he wrote, but "will appear to such as consider it without prejudice a great thing." Men who prefer "the observation of their laws, and their religion toward God, before the preservation of themselves and their country" deserve "a great many encomiums."

What do you have to believe about the Sabbath to be willing to die for it? Considering it a preferable form of social organization clearly won't suffice. Even perceiving it as a gift from God wouldn't seem to be enough, since life—creation—is also God's gift, so that when you die for the Sabbath you are simply trading one gift for another. Some historians of the Maccabean period interpret the Asidoi's religious intransigence as a form of class warfare. The country Jews resented the city Jews because the city Jews had access to élite Hellenistic institutions, such as gymnasiums and schools. So the country Jews took a radical stand against the city Jews, denouncing them as impious and unclean and becoming fanatical themselves. This explanation has a certain contemporary appeal. When you look at the events of our age, you can see how class resentment might merge with theology to form a glorified ideology of suicide.

But it also seems clear that these pious Jews brought a new intensity to the idea of the Sabbath itself. The seventh day was holy not just because God chose to rest on it; it was holy because it affirmed the divine order. It promised those who kept it that there *was* order rather than chaos. The future of the world depended on getting that order right.

Like Hamlet, the Asidoi felt that they lived in a time that was out of joint. It was during this era that the Jews invented another genre: the apocalyptic. In books such as Daniel and Enoch, also written in the time of Antiochus Epiphanes, angels revealed themselves in dreams and told tales of bloody wars of redemption. When would God make the time right again? Soon, the angels said. Daniel had a vision of a beast with teeth made of iron, nails of brass, and ten horns on his head. This image represented an evil kingdom out of which a king would arise who would "speak great words against the most High, and . . . think to change times and laws." Opposing them would be righteous men, and wise teachers, who would die by the sword. But the end of time would come, and then—in the very first reference we have to resurrection and judgment—"many of them that sleep in the dust of the earth shall awake, some to everlasting life, and some to shame and everlasting contempt."

It is thought that Daniel's "wise teachers"—whether historical personages or poetic longings—inspired the Asidoi to go down into the caves and die on the Sabbath. If the Asidoi read Daniel literally, which they probably did, they believed that if they died while keeping the Sabbath, the end of time would come and they would rise again.

Even if their faith was less scripturalist than that, they felt that to keep the Sabbath was to assert that time had a beginning, a middle, and an end. Along with the apocalyptic, the ancient Israelites also invented the idea of a history moving toward a divine end—toward the establishment of God's kingdom on earth. "They had learned from the Bible," Yosef Yerushalmi writes, "that the true pulse of history often beat beneath its manifest surfaces." But you couldn't keep believing in God's time if you didn't remind yourself of it every week. If you forgot that time has a pattern, you might forget that history has one, too, and you would despair in the face of conquest, massacre, destruction; you'd start to doubt that the Babylonians, or the Assyrians, or the Romans were instruments of God's wrath; you'd start thinking that your suffering had no meaning.

It is no coincidence that many apocalyptic ways of dating the moment of redemption have a cosmic week—a seven—in them somewhere. Seven was a number pregnant with God's presence. A few centuries later, the Jewish philosopher Philo would argue that seven is the most perfect number, not just in God's mind but in nature as well. In the apocalyptic numerology, God would reappear and set the world to rights in seven ages, or in seventy weeks, or in seven thousand years. In keeping the Sabbath no matter what, you signaled your willingness to wait for that moment.

7.

A DECADE AFTER I went to summer camp, I went to college. I should say, I went to Yale. It's important to say that not only because I still have to fight a bad habit many Yalies fall into, which is to mumble the name, or to say, with supremely false modesty, "in New Haven," when asked where they go or went to school. It's also important because only at Yale in the 1980s could I have become a member of a new religion. The church of my sect was a modest colonial rectangle on a quiet patch of grass in the shadow of the neo-Gothic Old Campus. This was the comparative-literature department. Its charismatic leader was another proud murmurer, a Belgian with an old-world gentleness and remoteness of manner. This was Paul de Man.

I came to comparative literature from classics, where I had no business being, not having studied Latin and Greek in high school. After semesters and summers of trying to keep pace with boarding-school graduates who sang out their Latin and Greek like dons-in-training, and slogging through pages of Virgil and Homer each night when just to parse a line could take me an hour, I was relieved to take a literary-theory class in which intellectual success was measured out in brilliant or at least clever acts of mind, not philological mastery, and social success in degrees of sartorial and intellectual sophistication, and every paper seemed like a gleeful attack on exactly the sort of grim, grinding, grammatical puzzles I'd been struggling to solve for two years.

It was a good time to be a deconstructionist at Yale. De Man had cancer but was still among us, and his 1941 essay in a Belgian newspaper calling for a "solution" to the "Jewish problem" and an end to the "Semitic interference" in Western literature had not yet come to light. Literary theory still held the answer to everything, and attracted the brightest graduate students in the country. De Man's classes were hushed and reverential; he was dying, and we knew it, and prepared for class as if we were dying alongside him, starved for his thin smile of approval, his quiet nod to continue. We waited for him to unfold poems like pieces of origami. He and the French philosopher Jacques Derrida and the critics of the Yale School (Geoffrey Hartman, J. Hillis Miller, Harold Bloom) had revealed the volatile core of insta-bility and indeterminacy lurking underneath every philosophical as-sertion, every scientific method, every work of literature. Nothing we'd learned (we learned) meant what it claimed to mean. All texts were allegories of their own blindness. They glossed over the un-thinkable. Our job was to think it for them. We would turn rhetoric against literature and literature against everything else, and come up with something cold and pure and undeluded.

All this gave me an unusually palpable sense of purpose. I was a mole burrowing under the foundations of the tottering edifice of Knowledge. I hung out in the underground undergraduate library, so much uglier and friendlier than the classics library, all bright lights and stale air and soft-cushioned sectional sofas, and read the authors of the new canon: Nietzsche, Heidegger, Rousseau, Freud, Baudelaire.

I read the French feminists, too, and learned about the provisionality of identity. My identity had always felt pretty provisional to me, and now it turned out to be a social construct, not a biological fact or a matter of inheritance. My womanhood was an effect of material signifiers—lipstick, hairstyles, clothes—and literary and cultural texts that, in the interests of hegemonic power, denied me, suppressed me, objectified me, and shoehorned me into false binary oppositions, such as the opposition of sensuousness to reason, heterosexuality to homosexuality. "I" was a performance, not an essence, although in the labyrinthine world of campus politics this was a tricky distinction: I knew several undergraduate staffers at the Yale Women's Center who were busily discovering their essential lesbian selves, and others who were very performatively declaring themselves "political lesbians"— lesbians for all intents and purposes, that is, except in the apparently non-essential matter of sexual desire.

Not that any of this solved the basic problem of what to do about my life, particularly my romantic life. If femininity was nothing more than a performance, then appearances mattered more than ever— were all that mattered, really—and being successfully feminine required an even fiercer commitment than I'd ever managed to make to the art of self-presentation: to fashion, hair, weight loss, and, for a would-be female graduate student in comparative literature, the exact right mix of sweetness and knowingness. Far from liberating me, feminist theory was making me more self-conscious than ever.

One aspect of my self that was starting to seem usable, though, was my Jewishness, which I had refused to think about once my bat mitzvah was over. Jewishness was hot. Jewish writers and thinkers— Kafka, Paul Celan, Emmanuel Levinas—had been reconfigured as deconstructionist precursors. Graduate students were parsing rabbinical texts to learn the rabbis' playful approach to interpretation, their Walter Benjamin–like appreciation for the fragment, their disregard for the plain sense of texts. During my senior year, the French filmmaker Claude Lanzmann, who was doing the final cut of his nine-hour

Holocaust movie, *Shoah,* visited Yale from Paris, and one of my professors made his interviews with camp survivors the main text for her class on psychoanalytic theory. Geoffrey Hartman was starting a video archive of Holocaust testimonies and was editing a volume of critical studies of midrash, to which Derrida would contribute.

Meanwhile, I started dating an Orthodox graduate student. Or rather, I should say, I was dated by him, since our romance, such as it was, was largely a product of his energy. Harold Bloom, a powerful reader of mystical and heretical Jewish texts, had taught us to be suspicious of "normative" Judaism, but that wasn't a concern for me, because I was only playing along, an accidental, undercover anthropologist.

Philip—I'll call him—was a *ba'al teshuvah,* a born-again Jew. I registered him at first only as a misfit seeking the company of other misfits, such as—I figured that he figured—me. He was a physics geek, smart and round and sweaty and abrupt. I can't remember how we met or what exactly we did in the early phase of our relationship, though I recall a lot of coffee being drunk in the underground library's cafeteria, otherworldy because lit almost entirely by vending machines. We didn't go out on dates. He asked a lot of questions, and I gave a lot of answers. It was, I think, an interview. Once I met Philip's criteria, we moved quickly to the next phase of the operation, which was spending Shabbat together.

"Together" is the wrong word, actually. It's not as if I was going to stay with him. He drove me to the home of some friends of his in Westville, a neighborhood in northwest New Haven where many Orthodox Jews lived, and left me there. He then went to stay with another friend nearby. My hosts were very normal and very nice. The father of the family was another bearded *ba'al teshuvah,* a graduate of our school, pleasingly formal in his white shirt and black pants. His wife was sweet-faced, Orthodox-born and -educated, and her headscarf and long skirt had an odalisque sensuality. I remember three daughters, the oldest being about nine; there may have been a baby. The girls followed me around in happy astonishment, delighted to discover someone in greater need of correction than themselves. I could sing the blessing over the candles, but when I went to the bathroom I tore the toilet paper, a mysteriously forbidden act. I nearly began eating without waiting for the blessing—less out of ignorance than nerves. The following morning, I brushed my teeth with toothpaste and applied lipstick, two more mysterious violations of etiquette. The girls asked me repeatedly to reassure them that my parents were Jewish. They made a big show of trying to parse the categorical error that I represented: a Jew with no idea how to conduct herself on Shabbat.

Dinner was an exercise in successful cliché. There was the authentic version of everything that had been pallidly alluded to on my family's Shabbat table. The dining room was ablaze with candles, one for each member of the family and a pair just for me. My hostess waved her hands enigmatically in the air and covered her eyes before saying the blessing. There was a two-handled laver and a basin for washing the hands before saying the blessing over the challah. There was a smell of braised meat. Sabbath songs were droned in a minor key throughout the meal. Crystal bowls of candy had been put out for snacking before dessert. Philip dropped me off and left for synagogue with his friend; my hostess and her children and I dressed, lit the candles, then, after the men returned, stood at attention during the blessings. Then the meal was served. I was glad to be a stranger in this particular strange land, I thought, because as a woman I had the option of hiding behind the gestures of female obligation. I could help lay out the silverware, carry in the food, clear the table, wash the dishes.

Except that I was never allowed to. My hostess deflected almost every offer to help. Her children could set the table, she said. She let other female guests clear, but when I tried to help she shooed me away with a friendly laugh. I slunk embarrassed back to the realm of the men, where my host was teaching some piece of Torah that I didn't understand.

It took me decades to understand that I had entered a domain so defamiliarized that I had to be maneuvered carefully around it, like a space alien likely to smash the furniture. The thirty-nine *melachot* and

the rabbinic add-ons ramify throughout a Sabbath-observant household, transmogrifying the performance of the most apparently simple
tasks. Most people have heard of the rules about not turning on lights
or stoves or electrical appliances, but fewer understand that when an
Orthodox Jew clears the table on the Sabbath she won't sort the
dishes by size, lest she perform the *melachah* of sorting. When she
washes the dishes, she'll wash only those she needs later in the day; the
others she will set aside or, if that means they'll turn foul, rinse. She
won't use a sponge, a scouring pad, or a dishtowel, lest she perform
the *melachah* of wringing. She will use only one of those nylon pads
with big fibers, or a nylon bottle brush. She may refuse to scour con-
gealed grease, lest she violate the rabbinic edict against *molid,* making
a new substance by changing something from one state to another. If
she dries a dish, she will hang up the towel, not squeeze it out. When
she wipes down the tablecloth, she will blot a spill, not scrub it out,
lest she wring or launder, another *melachah.*

When I learned this last rule, I finally understood the plastic
tablecloth, white and embossed with a floral motif, so seemingly out
of place in this elegant, faintly Central European household. Every
corner of the house offered up a puzzle that only further study would
solve: the bathrooms with the torn stacks of toilet paper (lest you tear)
and the absence of toothpaste (lest you smooth, a further refinement
on the *melachah* of scraping), the bedrooms with Scotch-taped outlets
(lest you kindle), the desks void of pens and scissors (lest you touch
muktzeh; that is, an object prohibited under rabbinic law because it
might lead to *melachot* such as writing and cutting).

The synagogue offered some respite from my mounting sense of
freakishness. I walked there with Philip—my hostess and her daughters having stayed home to prepare the house for the afternoon
luncheon—sat upstairs in the women's section, and hoped that no
one would notice my ignorance of the prayers. Not, I didn't know at
the time, that they would have cared if they did. Women don't have to
pray the same thrice-daily prayers that men do. They are not required
to say prayers at specific times because they're expected to submit to
the more open-ended temporal discipline of mothering. Had I read

Arendt by then, I would have had a theory to explain the difference between male and female behavior on the Sabbath. On Saturday, men cease from purposive, end-oriented endeavors. They free themselves to sing and drink and study Torah for the sake of studying Torah, *Torah lishmah*. They take action in the Arendtian sense of the term. They meet and greet and dispute. They fulfill their human potential. Women, on the other hand, do what they've been doing all week. They labor. They serve and clear and tuck the children into bed. They meet biological needs and provide emotional sustenance.

All this had more appeal than I felt it should have. I explained it to myself this way: My hostess could have pulled off her wig and become a doctor anytime she wanted to, so I didn't have to pity her. She had chosen her life, and since she had considerable personal authority she endowed it with a dignity I'd never perceived before. In Hebrew school I had learned that Judaism, as a religion, venerates the family; even if traditional Judaism doesn't grant women the power to study or lead services or do any of the things that give Jewish men honor in the eyes of other Jews, one day a week it honors the homes their wives make, the nourishment they provide, the bodies with which they make more bodies.

When I became a new mother myself, restricted to activities that could be synchronized with a baby's schedule, I began to see a genuine logic to this argument. That weekend, though, I thought of it as a rationalization against a much more powerful allure. I had never quite realized that there was a way to escape myself so ready to hand. I could just marry Philip and disappear into a long Sabbath afternoon! I could relinquish the overwhelming burden of being me and take up the lesser burden of being a member of a holy community. I could have my Jewish textuality and a sense of being right with the world, too.

That afternoon, Philip took me for a walk in a park. For the first time, he struck me as manly. I liked the way he steered me down the paths without touching me, a protective bulk of a man. I admired his mastery of the Orthodox idiom, the half-Yiddish of the *yeshiva bocher*. I half closed my eyes and squinted at the trees, imagining myself in something calf-length and woolen, him in a round fur hat and a long black suit. I made myself start an argument with him about whether separate spheres for the sexes were confining or liberating, and whether women should have the right to study Talmud. But my heart wasn't in it. His world was fixed and solid in ways mine wasn't. It made no sense to quibble with that. After Havdalah, Philip dropped me off at my apartment. He called the next day. I never called back.

PART FOUR

The Flight from Time

1.

A FEW CENTURIES AFTER THE DEATH OF THE ASIDOI, THERE AROSE A SAV-
ior in Israel. His name was Jesus.

By the time he appeared in the book in which we came to know
him—I am talking about the Gospel of Mark—he was already the
Messiah, the one destined to come at the end of the seven millennia
or aeons or days. Our first glimpse of Mark's Jesus has him being baptized in the wilderness while the Spirit of God descends and declares
him to be his son. Very shortly after that, Jesus does away with the
Sabbath.

You may wonder why I say the Gospel of Mark, since the Gospel
of Matthew precedes that of Mark in the New Testament. But Mark's
Jesus is older than Matthew's. Mark's gospel, written sometime be-
tween 68 and 73 C.E., cast the mold for the other Gospels. The
Gospels according to Matthew and Luke incorporated much of
Mark; the Gospel according to John came along a generation later.
Mark, in fact, probably invented the genre called "gospel," the quasi-
biographical novella offered up as an act of evangelical witnessing.
The real importance of Mark, though, is that he wrote a literary mas-

terpiece. His Jesus towers above the others, an abrupt, difficult man-god impatient with his disciples, secretive about his mission, and brimming with irresistible life. It is in Mark's Jesus that we feel the rough, uncanny power that inspired a new religion, rather than just a following.

Also remarkable is how much Mark makes of the Sabbath. No sooner does Mark's Jesus return from the wilderness than he strides into a synagogue in Capernaum during Sabbath services and drives a demon out of a man. It is his first miracle. His audience is stunned into silence, in part because the exorcism succeeds so well and in part because Jesus broke Sabbath law to perform it. Possession by a demon is a chronic condition and therefore something one should wait until the Sabbath is over to address. Jesus' disrespect for Sabbath law infuriates the Pharisees, the local religious leaders. (After the destruction of the Temple, the Pharisees evolved into what we call the rabbis, and they were very particular about their Sabbaths.)

The Pharisees start stalking Jesus, and soon enough they catch his disciples plucking grain on the Sabbath. He utters his aphorism: "The Sabbath was made for man, and not man for the Sabbath." And right after that, possibly even on the same Saturday, Jesus enters a synagogue and heals a man with a withered hand, another chronic condition that could have waited. At which point the Pharisees, who have begun muttering in dismay in the back of the room, step outside and set in motion the plot against Jesus that will ultimately result in his arrest and crucifixion.

Why does Mark care so much about the Sabbath? Don't be too distracted by the question of who Jesus "really" was and what he would have thought about the Sabbath. That someone named Jesus, Yehoshua, existed, that he had a message and a following and an effect on the world—historical evidence renders that fairly indisputable. It is probably safe to say that the historical Jesus would not have been dismissive of something as deeply woven into Jewish life as the Sabbath. The historical Jesus would have been a passionately religious Jew talking to other passionately religious Jews, or, more specifically, a Galilean talking openly to other Galileans and more cautiously to

Judeans. (Galileans were known for their folk piety, Judeans for their intellectual prowess and a certain condescension toward Galileans.)

That Jesus, if he raised the topic at all, would not have been making an argument *against* the Sabbath; he would have been taking a stand in the larger debate about what it meant to be a good Jew, with a corresponding opinion on the proper observance of the Sabbath. For that Jesus lived in a time of acute anxiety and extremes of behavior both religious and irreligious. The monkish Essenes in their desert communities forbade defecation on the Sabbath, while just up the road, in Jerusalem, Hellenizers blithely ignored the niceties of Sabbath boundaries. In between lay thousands of shades of ritual precision, with most people probably looking no further than their neighbors for guidance. When it came to the Sabbath, the historical Jesus would have had reform, not revolution, in mind. He was a Reform rabbi, not a Jew for Jesus.

But Mark was not talking about the historical Jesus. He was talking about the Christ, the anointed one, a hero in a cosmological drama. Mark doesn't explain Christ's attitude toward the Sabbath, but he does give hints in the way he tells his story. Of all the Gospel writers, Mark is the least patient. He moves his story along much more efficiently and economically than his counterparts do, and he says "immediately" a lot. The Greek word for "immediately," *euthys,* occurs fifty-one times in the New Testament; forty-one of those times are in Mark. John the Baptist dunks Jesus in the water, and the instant Jesus comes up—*euthys*—the heavens rip open and the Spirit descends like a dove from the sky. The Spirit tells Jesus that he is God's beloved son, and immediately casts him out into the wilderness. Jesus tells the fishermen Simon, Andrew, James, and John to follow him, and they do so immediately. The next thing you know, it's the Sabbath and they're barreling into the Capernaum synagogue and Jesus immediately begins to teach.

What follows is one of the most startling scenes in the New Testament, replete with "immediately"s. Not long after Jesus begins to speak, a man with "an unclean spirit"—that is, a demon or two— shouts him down, saying, "Let us alone; what have we to do with thee, thou Jesus of Nazareth? Art thou come to destroy us? I know thee who thou art, the Holy One of God."

"Shut up!" Jesus says to the demons—*phimotheti,* or "be muzzled," quite a rude expression in Greek; the King James Version renders it "Hold thy peace!"—and orders the spirits to leave the man. They do so promptly. Like the eyewitnesses, we readers are "all amazed," and, like them, we ask ourselves: Who were these demons who called Jesus by name? Why did they add, "Holy One of God"? How did Jesus *do* that? Or, as the Gospel puts it: "What thing is this? What new doctrine is this? For with authority commandeth he even the unclean spirits, and they do obey him." But there's no time for explanation. Word of Jesus' deeds ripples *immediately* across Galilee, and he has to cope with the vicissitudes of fame. By the time three stars have appeared in the sky, marking the end of the Sabbath, all the inhabitants of Capernaum have massed outside the house Jesus has retreated to and are demanding that he cure their sick and demented relatives.

We are still ten verses shy of the end of the first chapter of Mark. Mark is in a hurry, we realize, because Jesus is in a hurry. "Mark's Jesus is a man of action: dashing, busy, driven in rapid motion from synagogue to invalid, from shore to grainfield to sea," the historian Paula Fredriksen writes. Spiritually speaking, he's a shock trooper. He takes Galilee by surprise. As the demons suspect, he has come to destroy them, but by the time anyone else figures this out he has won his first battle. He has established a base camp on earth.

Or, as Harold Bloom puts it in an essay on Mark, "Apocalypse hovers." Joel Marcus, the editor of the Anchor Bible edition of Mark, uses the phrase "cosmic apocalyptic eschatological" to describe the kind of war that Mark's Jesus has come to fight. "Cosmic," because its scope comprises the heavens and the earth. "Apocalyptic," because Mark's gospel features epic battles between the forces of good and evil. "Cosmic apocalyptic": the entire cosmos has been captured by evil—by Satan and his demons—and requires liberation. And "eschatological," meaning "having to do with the end," because the final, transformative battle could occur at any minute. "Whether the Jewish War is ongoing or Jerusalem has already been destroyed, we are never told," Bloom says, "but Mark lives in what he believes to be the end-time."

In short, when Mark's Jesus bursts onto the stage like someone breaking through the back wall of a set, time itself changes. It speeds up. Jesus' arrival signals the beginning of the end. He operates within the compressed time frame that we now call a state of emergency. In an emergency, normal rules are suspended and new ones are devised. "The time is short," Paul will write to his followers in Corinth. Under the circumstances, who would expect Jesus to let the Sabbath slow him down?

But therein lies Jesus' problem. When he gets to the Capernaum synagogue, no one besides Satan, the disciples, and the demons knows what the circumstances are. It is up to Jesus to show the people who he is and what his coming means. So he must violate the Sabbath, and not only to defeat the demons. He has to get across, boldly and publicly, the novel notion that there *is* an emergency, and he has to convince his listeners that he has the authority to declare it.

The confrontation in the synagogue achieves both ends. Jesus gets up and, Mark says, speaks with authority. You have to understand this sentence in its technical sense: "Speaking with authority" would have meant breaking the well-known and firmly established rules of Jewish argumentation. According to these, a teacher advancing an interpretation of Scripture must invoke the authority of older interpreters in order to avoid appearing to make an original point, for to the Pharisaic mind *original* meant *unsubstantiated*. Mark never tells us *what* Jesus says, however, because the content of his speech doesn't matter. What matters is *how* Jesus says it. He speaks from his own authority, which upsets his listeners. Then he backs up his right to speak in this fashion with a show of uncanny power over demons. And he performs these acts on the Sabbath, an opportune time from his point of view, since it is the day of the week when the people gather together and make themselves available as witnesses.

Whatever the actual Jesus may or may not have thought of the Sabbath, the Pharisees of the Gospels do not misinterpret the Jesus of the Gospels when they suspect that he does not hold the Sabbath in as much esteem as they do. The Pharisees surrounded the Sabbath as if it were the Temple, with a series of protective fences. Mark's Jesus seems determined to knock those fences down. With the end so near, indeed already here, with the advent of a Messiah who is himself divine, *all* time is holy time. To deem one day holier than another is to make distinctions at a time and in a place where such distinctions have been rendered null and void. It is to demonstrate a spirit so narrow, so lacking in imagination and capaciousness, that it can't free itself from the past and move into the future.

By the end of the scene in the Capernaum synagogue, we have completed the transition into the apocalyptic mode. The hero—the deus ex machina—has made himself known in a leveling burst of glory. The moment is now. From here on in, the pace will be swift, the pitch operatic. Those who refuse to budge from these inert patches of time and space, from Sabbath and Temple, will never know the bliss of the promised end.

2.

TODAY, THE PACE of life has quickened even more dramatically than in the book of Mark, and larger-than-life superheroes race to narrative climaxes on every possible electronic platform. We live as Mark wrote, in a state of apocalyptic urgency. Relatively few of us believe that Jesus is about to return, but just over the horizon of waking life, in nightmares and disaster movies and science-fiction novels, visions of the end play themselves out—clashes of civilizations or meteorological convulsions or nuclear holocausts or financial catastrophe or some combination thereof. We attribute the swiftness with which life sweeps past us not to God and the forces of redemption but to social forces beyond our control. In our Durkheimian era, God is another word for the awesome power of organized collective entities.

If you want to blame something for the heavy, humiliating sense of time moving above and beyond our control, you should, as you already know, blame clocks. You should specifically blame railroad clocks. And wireless telegraphs. Fifteenth-century church clocks abstracted time into money; nineteenth-century railroad clocks abstracted local time into global time; but railroad clocks also synchronized schedules across vast swaths of terrain—mountains, plains, deserts, jungles, villages, and cities—thereby forcing the industrialized nations to standardize their systems of time measurement. And then, at the turn of the twentieth century, came the wireless telegraph with its magical instantaneity, which made the industrialized nations coordinate their time zones with one another, and then with the developing nations, making the reach of standard time truly global.

With this integration came simultaneity, the sense that thousands of events were taking place at once in thousands of places. People began to learn, first from the telegraph, then from radio, newsreels, television, and the Internet, that what was happening *now*, all over the globe, mattered more than what was happening *here*.

The communications scholar Manuel Castells talks about the "space of flows," which he contrasts with the "space of places." The space of flows is the space of the electronic circuits, nodes, and hubs that transmit the bytes that bind us together into social networks. The space of places is what the space of flows leaves behind—the decaying streets and buildings and bridges and cemeteries and rivers and oceans that used to mark the boundaries of our individual worlds.

Castells draws a similar contrast between what he calls "linear, irreversible, measurable, predictable time" and "timeless time." Linear time moves forward, proceeding according to a traditional and prescribed sequence of events. You are born. You grow up, get a job, marry, and have children. You acquire your storehouse of memories. Your children grow up and do the same. You retire. You die. In timeless time, the life cycle loses its familiar rhythms. Vacation times vary, as the blocks of leisure associated with summer give way to the new economy's need for flexible work schedules ("just-in-time labor"). Reproductive schedules vary. It is no longer necessary to give birth in the first half of your life; the fertility industry has made it possible for women to bear children after menopause. The age of death varies, and may one day be suspended indefinitely. Not that these gyrations in biological time are all bad. They may turn out to be liberating. After all, only malleable work schedules will allow women to remain in the workforce and care for their children in a manner acceptable to them.

Nevertheless, when you dissolve the old structures and boundaries of time—the calendar of holidays and festivals, the geographical distances, the chronobiological cycles—you remove the brakes that slow down the perpetual motion machine of postindustrial capitalism. Marx was the first to point out that divorcing time from context and commodifying it as money leads directly to temporal compression. When time is money, speed equals more of it. He who can make more of something in less time gets to slash prices or beat his competitor into stores, and he who can produce faster must, or risk going out of business when a competitor does it first. And when the market picks up the pace, so do our lives. Milestones skitter past us like videos in fast-forward: friendships and marriages form and dissolve; homes are bought and sold; jobs are taken and left. Death is no longer certain. Nor are taxes. The only thing that can be guaranteed is that long before we're ready, we—our professional know-how, our familiarity with the world, our sense of style—will have become obsolete.

We think of inevitable obsolescence as new, and certainly we grow obsolete faster than we used to, but the experience is old. Some poor soul from an ancien régime is always being left behind. Some poor rural Israelite is always feeling the anguish of watching her children seduced into new, gleaming gymnasiums and a new, faster, more cosmopolitan way of life. In *The Education of Henry Adams,* Henry Adams offers a snapshot of this eternally recurring process. Adams is describing "the law of acceleration" of progress, which, he says, speeded up to such a degree after 1900 that a person born in one generation could no longer learn anything worth knowing from a teacher born in the previous one. In the century leading up to 1900, there emerged a set of "supersensual forces," by which he meant steam power, gunpowder, electricity, instruments of measurement that far surpassed the capacities of the human senses. Before these vast engines, Adams says, "the man of science stood at first as bewildered and helpless as, in the fourth century, a priest of Isis before the Cross of Christ."

Adams's metaphor says a lot. Christ was not a "supersensual force" in the technological sense that Adams gave the term, nor did he change time as materially as the clock did. But he ushered in an intensified, quickened experience of time. The tragedy of Christ's death, coupled with the promise of his return, endowed the time in between—the *nun,* as it was called in Greek, or the now—with a previously unimaginable electricity. I call this time the superpresent. Christian theology distinguishes between two temporal orders: the time of *chronos,* the Greek word for "passing time," and the time of *kairos,* Greek for "moment of crisis." To convert to early Christianity would have been to plunge from *chronos* to *kairos,* from a life measured out in minute increments of ritual performance into the midst of one of the greatest dramas ever played out in cosmic history.

The literary critic Frank Kermode puts it this way: Once the Christ came along to redeem humankind and remedy the consequences of the Fall, "a new series of time began, and it was somehow, at least potentially, of a different quality; the Incarnation entailed the intervention of God into human time, after which nothing could be as it was." Paul made a similar point when he wrote to the Galatians about "the fulness of the time." The time is full, Paul explains, because it is the moment when God "sent forth his Son." Kierkegaard called the fullness of time "the pivotal concept in Christianity, that which made all things new." Paul endows this overplenitude with an aching sensuality. The fullness of time is the moment when God (through Christ and the Holy Spirit) invades the present and fills it with his presence.

Imagine how elating it must have been to convert to Christianity. You fled the bodily, the time-bound, that which was subject to decay; you were caught up in something bigger and swifter and more powerful than yourself. "Have you ever had a gallop on a horse?" asks the greatest of all Christian apologists, C. S. Lewis, in *The Lion, the Witch and the Wardrobe.* Lewis is describing Lucy and Susan's ride on the back of Aslan, the lion who represents Jesus in his allegorical Narnia series. "Think of that; and then take away the heavy noise of the hoofs and the jingle of the bits and imagine instead the almost noiseless padding of the great paws. Then imagine instead of the black and gray or chestnut back of the horse the soft roughness of the golden fur, and the mane flying back in the wind. And then imagine you are going about twice as fast as the fastest racehorse. But this is a mount that doesn't need to be guided and never grows tired. He rushes on and on, never missing his footing, never hesitating, threading his way with perfect skill between tree-trunks, jumping over bush and briar and the smaller streams, wading the larger, swimming the largest of all."

3.

HOW DO YOU EXPLAIN what time feels like to someone right out of college? I can only tell you what time felt like to me. It felt like a timed test that I was flunking.

I had discovered, at college, that there were people who seemed predestined to succeed, as if good fairies had granted success as their gift at their baptisms. I had had the vague idea that accomplishment was something you attained after serving a long apprenticeship at some difficult trade, years and years after college. But by the time I graduated, I understood that the future had long since arrived. Jodie Foster was in my class; she put on weight and looked deceptively like the rest of us, but she nonetheless moved in a much faster lane. I had classmates who had written novels and directed movies by the time they arrived, and still others (or the same ones) who had published their novels with respectable publishing houses, gotten deals with Hollywood, and launched magazines by the time they left.

These classmates went to New York, as I did. My friends and I were fact-checkers, production assistants, paralegals. They were editors, writers, nonprofit entrepreneurs. We ran into them at parties and tried to cloak envy in self-mocking wit. We were above all those books that promised success through effective time management, but whenever we could we sneaked peeks at them in the bookstore.

It was the late 1980s, the end of the Reagan administration and the ascendancy of the yuppie, and those of my classmates who hadn't found a perch on the fast track of a Hollywood studio had snagged jobs at Goldman Sachs or Citibank or McKinsey. I had grown up on the literature of countercultural, therapeutic self-actualization— Theodore Roszak and Herbert Marcuse and Norman O. Brown, those questers for ecstasy and authenticity and true selves—and felt stranded by my classmates and their carefully plotted plans, career ladders, salaries, bonuses, promotions. I found an apartment in Greenpoint, Brooklyn, which in the early nineties wasn't the hipster enclave it would later become. It was still Polish and poor, with row houses clad in aluminum siding and a main street, called Manhattan Avenue, packed with discount stores and dimly lit Cuban-Chinese and Polish restaurants. My apartment sat above a Chinese restaurant. I shared it with a fellow student, Sasha, from the graduate program in journalism that I had dropped out of. It was a strange apartment, with three shallow front rooms and no doors. We lived at opposite ends of the apartment, with no privacy from each other or from the outside world. We were too high up to be seen from the street; but for that, we might have been objects on display in a shop window.

But it was light and cheap and only half an hour from the East Village. We liked the shouts and honks of Manhattan Avenue. It suited our sense of being transient and public, exposed to the wave patterns of some higher, faster, not quite visible flux. We ate takeout from cheap Polish cafeterias; we drank in Polish bars; we went to parties thrown by people on the art scene that was just emerging in Williamsburg. We walked down the dark, empty cobblestoned street over which loomed shuttered warehouses and the old Domino factory. We thought of ourselves as tourists, though the locals must have seen us as something much more dangerous, as gentrifiers. They were right, but wrong. We didn't want to burrow in and make Greenpoint our home. We were busy. We had to maximize our potential; we had to make good on our promise. The first day of every month, I walked down to the second floor and gave our landlady the rent check with a twinge of shame. She spoke no English, but if she could have, I thought she'd say, "What? You still here?"

I tried to make the time pay, but with little result. I had a half-formed notion that I should be a producer of culture, perhaps in the film industry, maybe on the business side. Not that I cared a whit about the business side. I thought that knowing how money worked would give me the leverage to make Great Art. I was an assistant at a distribution company that marketed foreign films. I was a production assistant on a television shoot. I did secretarial work for a feminist filmmaker in a huge, messy loft in SoHo. I wrote press releases for an avant-garde film collective in Tribeca.

Since then I have read many sociological studies of alienated, un-employed, unrealistic youth, probably because I recognize in them versions of myself, odious as that comparison is, given their infinitely less privileged backgrounds and their complete lack of options and safety nets. In one such study, a sociologist contrasted young people who take *time out*—that is, postpone their career or education in order to enrich themselves—and those who *drop out,* or fall off the train of productive, career-building moving-toward-the-future time. One dropout in the study, Linda, spoke of becoming a nurse's assistant but did nothing to achieve that goal. Time was not real to her. She felt de-tached from it, uprooted, and that made her feel unreal, too. The days floated past her meaninglessly, and nothing that happened in the pres-ent seemed to bear any relationship to the future, which existed in its own contained imaginary bubble.

I felt what she felt, even though I was not a dropout. Time was unreal to me. It passed, but overhead, with a *whoosh* like Aslan. Time never entered my body; it was never anything that I could grab hold of. I lived shamefully outside its rules, outside its limits, beyond its boundaries. I wanted to bring about an end to this dreary sense of time moving beyond my control, but I felt too weightless to change. If the Christian kind of timelessness lifted you above time, this kind dropped you outside it. My job interviews generally ended as I imag-ine Linda's did. Employers would ask me to explain myself, and I would speak quickly and fluently about my goals at *that* point and *that* point and why I'd done *that,* but in the end I could not make my story make sense. I usually ended up kicking my legs in my chair like a five-year-old.

Meanwhile, I moved a lot. I moved from Greenpoint to a room

on the top floor of a brownstone in Park Slope, then to an apartment on the north side of the Slope, called Prospect Heights. I had no idea why I kept moving. I knew that I wanted to stay in Brooklyn. It seemed to me that it still had something to say to me, something I hadn't heard yet. I loved its decrepit brownstones, shuttered warehouses, polluted sea vistas, ethnic neighborhoods. Riding through Brooklyn on my bicycle, I imagined I was Walt Whitman on an epic American perambulation.

What was I looking at? A preference evolved for neighborhoods where the people came from somewhere else. I looked for store signs in foreign languages, preferably in foreign alphabets—Greek, Russian, Arabic, Hebrew. I circled around churches, the onion-domed Eastern Orthodox ones, the storefront mosques in Cobble Hill, the black Baptist churches with the strangely Jewish names. Eventually, I narrowed my focus to neighborhoods with signs in Hebrew and Yiddish. I rode up and down Ocean Parkway, studying the giant letters above the grand synagogues and yeshivot that lined the service roads of the elegant boulevard. I stared hungrily at the women in their wigs and long skirts and cheap, sensible shoes, the men with their hats and fringes.

A few months before I moved out of my Greenpoint apartment, Sasha had moved back to Manhattan, and I had taken in the friend of a friend, a West German law student named Maria, who was doing a summer internship at the United Nations. She taught me rudimentary German in partial lieu of rent. When she went back to West Berlin, I visited her once, and from then on I went back every year. She shared her apartment in what was then the bohemian neighborhood of Kreuzberg with Anna, a graduate student in Jewish studies; to my surprise, this was an increasingly popular field of study in West Germany, and one that proceeded in the total absence of Jewish students. Anna had a boyfriend named Klaus, a recent Ph.D., who used to lecture me on the contents of the Jewish siddur, or prayer book. Once we went to Yom Kippur services together in a newly reopened synagogue in what had been East Berlin, and he expressed surprise at my ignorance of the fine points of the holiday and its liturgy. I was

embarrassed and resentful. How dare this German one-up me Jew-
ishly?

Nonetheless, I became closer to Anna and Maria's friends than to
my own, which is how it happened that one day years later I found
myself, along with an American friend equally obsessed with matters
German, showing New York to a group of women from the former
East Germany who had come to explain the advantages of Communist day-care policies to a conference on women and law. We asked
them what they wanted to see first, and they said Borough Park in
Brooklyn, which has one of the densest concentrations of visibly Orthodox Jews outside Israel. The women wanted to buy fancy hats,
they told us, and there were plenty of those to be found in Orthodox
Jewish neighborhoods, since married women who live there are
obliged to cover their heads. My friend and I looked at each other. I
felt a stab of dislike. Under the roar of the subway, I murmured to my
friend that we were off to go "Juden-gucken," which means, literally,
"Jew-peeping" but if said a certain way sounds, in English, like "Jew-
cooking."

But that's what I'd been doing: Jew-peeping. And I did it most
often on Saturdays, when the men wore their silk stockings and round
fur hats and the women, too, wore their best dresses and hats. I circled
back and back upon the neighborhoods. I was aware of violating their
Sabbath space with my bicycle shorts and my bare shoulders, but I felt
protected by my nakedness, too. It made me feel safe, unseen.

Years later, I saw an exhibition of paintings by the German Ex-
pressionists known as Die Brücke, a group of male art and architecture students who greeted the turn of the twentieth century with a
classic fit of art-school bad-boy attitude. They borrowed Cézanne's
fascination with the primitive—with Negroes, Samoans, full-lipped
and full-breasted female nudes—but, lacking his age and wisdom and
depth, also lacked his knack for jolting figures into our line of vision
as fully spatial, non-objectified, *living* bodies. The primitives of the
Die Brücke painters were flat stabs at something, expressions of a
longing to escape to another world. They made no connection. I felt
a sick wave of self-recognition. I had looked at the Jewish bodies the

way these German painters had looked at their models' black and brown and female ones—with hunger, envy, pity, horror, and a secret self-satisfaction at my daring. I never got off my bicycle and talked to the objects of my gaze. You speak to them, I thought, and they see right through you. They know you for the tourist you are.

It was my best friend from high school who got me to enter a synagogue. The daughter of a Lutheran minister, and a pianist and poet, she moved in with me in Park Slope during a short-lived tryout of life in New York City and went to church every Sunday. At one point I asked if I could go with her, and she very sweetly said no. In retrospect, I can't blame her. I must have been a turbulent presence.

Around that time, though, a movie titled *A Stranger Among Us* came out. It starred Melanie Griffith as a policewoman who goes undercover, implausibly, in a Hasidic community in Brooklyn. She even attends services with her so-called family. The synagogue was a picture postcard of old-world Jewry, with a bimah, or raised altar, in the middle of the room and a women's balcony. The scene, I read in the local press, had been filmed at a non-Orthodox synagogue down the block. Its interior turned out to be as detail-rich as its exterior was blank. When the film crew came, they built the old-fashioned central altar, replaced the old chandeliers with less modern ones, brought out some pews that had been hidden in the basement, and scrubbed everything till it had the requisite spiritual gleam.

I went in one Saturday. There were the wooden pews, though the altar had been taken down; the stained-glass windows; the bronze *ner tamid,* or "eternal light," hanging before the ark of the Torah. I sat in a pew at the back of the sanctuary, thoroughly amused by the Disneyfication of my ancestral architecture, the sheer artificiality of it all, and burst into tears.

The rabbi at the synagogue was not a gregarious man. He never came over and put a hand on my shoulder or asked me what was the matter. Nor did anyone else. I went back the following week, and was left alone again. I did this week after week. I must have been emitting radio waves of discomfort, because it was months before anyone invited me home for lunch after services, and more than a year before I began, tentatively, to join a Sabbath community. I was glad to be left alone, and not sure that I wanted friendship. I was a fraud, an impostor, a cliché. I did not want to be acknowledged. And yet, perversely—and even though I've always disliked the word *spiritual,* which seems a way of averting the eyes from the accusatory glare of the holy—I sometimes think that those sad, solitary Sabbaths were the most spiritual I've ever had.

4.

THE CHRISTIAN NOTION of the holy life as a flight from earthly bonds reflected another shift: from the rule-bound, or "bureaucratic," community to a "charismatic" one. The terms are Max Weber's, and he takes Christ as the very model of the charismatic leader, the figure who dissolves existing hierarchies and laws and runs society on the strength of personal authority alone. Christ's authority came from his genius for quickening spirits, not from his mastery of a method or rules or a body of knowledge.

Jesus came with his charisma to liberate the world from the tyranny of the law, that harsh and petty "schoolmaster," as Paul put it. Actually, Paul probably only said "custodian," a much less negative term, and meant that Jesus liberated *Gentiles* from the law, not Jews, and he may not have found the law particularly tyrannical for those who were born into it, as he had been. The church fathers who came after him, however, removed as they were from the Jewish matrix of beliefs, thought he was throwing out the Mosaic Code for everybody, for all time, and that is the view of Paul and the law that has prevailed ever since. By this reading, Paul said that Jewish law existed only to oppress all of humankind with its exacting standards, to drive us to despair and thus into the arms of Christ. Before there were the restrictions and complications of holy law, there was Abraham's simplicity of faith.

Paul's critique of Jewish law, even in its most limited form, had everything to do with the ethnic politics of the Jesus movement. It began as an observant Jewish sect but almost immediately tumbled outside the borders of Palestine into a much less Jewish world. Not that Jesus' followers thereby entered a wholly Gentile world. Scholars of late antiquity make clear that the cities outside Palestine in which Christianity blossomed, such as, say, Antioch, Rome, and Alexandria, possessed large, diverse Jewish communities. These, though minorities in an age lacking any concept of minority rights, were often blessed with political power, or had at least worked out an arrangement with the local authorities. As Christianity moved outside Palestine, it established itself on the edges of these communities. But it also drew followers from among the surprisingly large cohort of Gentile friends and neighbors who were attracted to monotheism and the high moral standards of Judaism. These adherents may have studied Torah or kept the Sabbath, but they weren't ready or willing to shoulder the entire yoke of Jewish law. Nonetheless, synagogue records throughout the ancient diaspora reveal that significant numbers of these fellow travelers attended services or associated in some other way with the synagogue.

Christ's evangelists baptized their way through the ranks of the sympathizers, but over time they met with increasing success among non-sympathizing Gentiles. This raised the question of whether or not the converts to Christianity ought to adopt all the customs that made the Jew seem so peculiar—objectionable, really—to Gentile observers. Should the new Christians be circumcised, abstain from pork, halt work on the Sabbath?

Such questions rubbed the early Christian psyche at its most sensitive spot. Day after day, the converts of Rome, Asia Minor, and the West were required to account for themselves. Who were these zealous, often ill-educated people? Why did they follow a Jewish preacher who had been hung up on a cross, of all the ignominious ways to die? Were they Jews, Gentiles, or neither? Clearly, they had joined some sort of minority. But was it a spiritual élite, as they claimed, or a rabblement of heretics and outcasts, a minority of a minority, as many Jews and Gentiles declared?

It is never easy to move through the world unsure of oneself, but the quest for Christian identity must have been particularly unsettling. Conversion from one communal affiliation to another was not unheard of in the ancient world—many Judeophiles, for instance, wound up becoming Jews—but it remained the exception. Becoming a Christian back then demanded a much greater tolerance for social dislocation than it does today, because it meant leaving the known order of things and entering into an as yet unmapped society. Religious beliefs were inherited, not chosen. "What we now think of as 'religion' had a clear genealogical nexus then," Paula Fredriksen writes. "People worshipped the gods native to them. To undergo a rite that would turn a pagan into a Jew would make as little sense to most pagans as would a modern person's undergoing a ritual by which she would somehow be transformed from being, say, actually culturally English to actually culturally Italian."

Besides, whatever the Greeks and the Romans may have thought of the Jews (and some evinced mild admiration, though more expressed disdain), they respected antiquity and sneered at innovation. The second-century philosopher Celsus, for instance, was no fan of Jews, but he had even less patience for Christians, whom he called failed Jews. They got a basic Jewish concept—monotheism—wrong, and they worshipped a man who had been crucified like a common criminal. "You make yourself a laughing-stock in the eyes of everybody," Celsus wrote, "when you blasphemously assert that the other gods made manifest are phantoms, while you worship a man who is more wretched than even what really are phantoms, and who is not even any longer a phantom, but in fact dead."

And yet cutting ties to families and the past is what the Christ of the Gospels demanded of his followers. He set the example by refusing to recognize his mother and brother when they asked to speak to him, saying that his followers made up all the family he needed: " 'Who is my mother? And who are my brethren?' And he stretched forth his hand toward his disciples, and said, 'Behold my mother and my brethren! For whosoever shall do the will of my father which is in heaven, the same is my brother, and sister, and mother.' "

Paul grappled nonstop with the problem of Christian identity. So did those who came after him. The popular Gnostic leader Marcion, writing in the middle of the second century, found *all* Jewish aspects of Christianity repugnant, and tried to expel the Old Testament from the canon of Christian books. The church fathers thought this excessively anti-Jewish and called it heresy. The Ebionite Christians, on the other hand, followed the Mosaic Code, keeping the Sabbath on Saturday and other laws well into the fourth century. That degree of inclusiveness veered too close to Judaism, and it, too, was deemed heretical.

Paul preached to the Gentiles, mostly in Asia Minor, until his death sometime between 64 and 67 C.E. He intervened frequently in disputes about Jewish observance. His main opponent in this debate was Jesus' brother James, the head of a church in Jerusalem that continued to follow Mosaic Law. Paul worked out his answers to James's challenges in a series of gorgeously argued letters to Christian communities outside Palestine. His supple prose style gives these letters a richness and an elusiveness rarely found in the history of epistolary writing, and debates about what he meant to say—and particularly about what he was trying to say about Judaism and the Jews—are, if anything, more intense than ever before, the Holocaust having made early-Christian anti-Judaism seem more suspect than ever before.

If you had to reduce Paul's magnificently worded and carefully hedged theological edifice to one crude assertion, it would be that Jesus erased all distinctions between Jew and non-Jew, holy and unholy, at least insofar as those distinctions dictated who would be saved and who would not at the end of time. In other words, Paul invented a kind of universalism—you could call it end-time universalism. Confined as it was to the postapocalyptic moment, this universalism still represented an erosion of ancient boundaries, and from this erosion of boundaries flows much of what is radical in Paul's thought. For if there is to be no difference, at the end of days, between Jew and non-Jew, then there will no longer be any need for the Law; and if there is to be no need for the Law, then there will be no means of differentiating between the sacred and the profane; and if there is no longer to be any way to distinguish the holy from the unholy, then everything will have been made holy through Jesus' death and through his grace.

And if all will have been made holy, then ultimately all hierarchical systems of social valuation will become meaningless. That, at least, is how I read the verse from Paul's epistle to his followers in Galatia: "There is neither Jew nor Greek, there is neither bond nor free, there is neither male nor female: for ye are all one in Christ Jesus."

From Paul's desire to clarify the status of Gentile converts comes the revolutionary inclusiveness that endows Christianity with its irrepressible buoyancy. And what Paul's Christianity liberated Gentile Christians from is, among other things, the Sabbath. For, in Paul's opinion, only Christ could sanctify time. In his letter to the Galatians, Paul chides them for observing "days, and months, and times, and years." He writes: "After that ye have known God, or rather are known of God, how turn ye again to the weak and beggarly elements, whereunto ye desire again to be in bondage?" By "elements," Paul meant the movements of the heavenly bodies, by which both pagans and Jews determined their holy times. Christ, he was saying, mooted such earthbound ways of determining holiness, at least for Gentiles. He had freed his followers from the sclerotic Sabbath laws like a Moses of the overregulated soul, facing down Pharisees and priests much as the son of Hebrews confronted Pharaoh. (It doesn't hurt that *Pharisees* sounds a lot like *Pharaoh*.)

5.

IT WAS IGNATIUS, the bishop of Antioch under the Roman emperor Trajan at the very beginning of the second century C.E., who came up with the term "Sabbatizing." It echoed another term, "Judaizing." Both terms gave voice to the feeling that it was absurd to adhere to Jewish law in a post-Jewish age. The second-century Roman defender of the faith, Justin Martyr, told a Jew named Trypho, with whom he supposedly debated, that God gave the Jews the Sabbath to punish them—"because of your sins and your hardness of heart." Justin reasoned from Scripture: Since God loved Noah, Abraham, Isaac, Jacob, and Joseph, and none of *them* kept the Sabbath, God must have imposed the burden of the Sabbath to make the Jews pay for the sin of worshipping the golden calf. Or, as Justin tells Trypho, "you Jews" demonstrated your innate nature as "a ruthless, stupid, blind, and lame people, children in whom there is no faith." In much the same way, God gave circumcision to the Israelites to set them apart from the other nations of the earth. The purpose of these unwholesome customs, Justin declared, "was that you and only you might suffer the afflictions that are now justly yours; that only your lands be desolate, and your cities ruined by fire; that the fruits of your land be eaten by strangers before your very eyes."

The Alexandrian Barnabas, also writing in the second century, thought that Jewish rituals, including the Sabbath, were simple misinterpretations of God's intent. The physical commandments, Barnabas maintained, were allegories. The most vivid illustration of Barnabas's spiritualizing hermeneutics can be seen in his discussion of kashruth. Why, asked Barnabas, did Moses say, " 'Thou shall eat neither swine, nor eagle, nor hawk, nor crow, nor any fish that has no scales on it' "? Barnabas explained: When Moses prohibited eating swine, he *really* meant to tell the Jews to avoid consorting with people who are swinelike, in that their urge to satisfy their hunger drives out every nobler sentiment. The eagle, the hawk, and the raven are predators; likewise, said Barnabas, one should avoid not the flesh of those birds but the company of men like them, "such people as do not know how to obtain their food by sweat and labor, but, in their disregard for law, plunder other people's property." And on Barnabas went, a Christian Aesop, reinterpreting every animal whose flesh is prohibited by Jewish law as a miniature moral fable.

As for the Sabbath, Barnabas said it should not be seen as the seventh day of the week; rather, it should be seen as the seventh day of Creation, and also as the seventh millennium, that end of time in which God's son—Jesus, of course—would arrive and destroy a wicked age.

Why did the Jews fail to understand their own prophet's metaphors? It was not given to them to understand. As Barnabas put it, the Jews circumcised their bodies, not their ears.

6.
___

IF THE CHRISTIANS OBJECTED to the Sabbath, how did they fix on Sunday? We don't really know. The New Testament gives no answer. It furnishes no evidence of a regular Sunday gathering other than a handful of references to the day that *can* be interpreted as indicating that it had been singled out in some fashion—though only if you're willing to ignore alternate readings that suggest that Sunday was just one day among others. Not until the second century do we find Sunday described as a day when Christians gather to worship. Ignatius, Barnabas, and Justin all allude to it. Justin writes:

> And on the day called Sunday there is a meeting in one place of those who live in cities or the country, and the memoirs of the apostles or the writings of the prophets are read as long as time permits. When the reader has finished, the president in a discourse urges and invites [us] to the imitation of these noble things. Then we all stand up together and offer prayers. And, as said before, when we have finished the prayer, bread is brought, and wine and water, and the president similarly sends up prayers and thanksgivings to the best of his ability, and the congregation assents, saying the Amen; the distribution, and reception of the consecrated [elements] by each one, takes place and they are sent to the absent by the deacons. Those who prosper, and who so wish, contribute, each one as much as he chooses to. What is collected is deposited with the president, and he takes care of orphans and widows, and those who are in want on account of sickness or any other cause, and those who are in bonds, and the strangers who are sojourners among [us], and, briefly, he is the protector of all those in need. We all hold this common gathering on Sunday, since it is the first day, on which God transforming darkness and matter made the universe, and Jesus Christ our Saviour rose from the dead on the same day. For they crucified him on the day before Saturday, and on the day after Saturday, he appeared to his apostles and disciples and taught them these things which I have passed on to you also for your serious consideration.

The order of the Sunday service evolved sometime between the ministry of Christ in the early thirties of the first century and the middle of the second, when Justin would have been writing. The Christian world at that point consisted of small groups scattered across Asia Minor and Europe, some buried deep within cities, some little more than house churches, many cut off from the others, and each with its own idiosyncratic syncretism—its mix of Jewishness, paganness, and "Christianness." Each community's rituals reflected the backgrounds of its members and the personalities of its founders. Jewish Christians may have gone to synagogues on the Sabbath and worshipped on Sunday, too, while pagan Christians may have stopped observing the Sabbath, or at least stayed away from synagogues, but they may not have singled out Sunday, either.

One student of Sunday, Willy Rordorf, thinks that the earliest Christians in Jerusalem began the tradition of gathering on Sunday in honor of Christ's Resurrection, which happened on the first day of the week. Another scholar of Sunday, Samuele Bacchiocchi, argues that the shift from Saturday to Sunday happened a century later, in Rome, where Gentiles predominated, and where Jews had become a vilified enemy after the Jewish Revolt against Roman rule, quashed in 132 C.E. Bacchiocchi (a Seventh-Day Adventist, which means that he objects to the switch from Saturday to Sunday) points out that around the time Justin was writing, a new custom arose in Christian Rome: the Saturday fast. Nothing could be less like a Jewish Sabbath celebration than a fast, so, Bacchiocchi reasons, the fast must have been intended to heighten the contrast between Jews and Christians and to make Sunday look more appealing.

One thing we do know is what Sunday was not. It was not a day of rest. The realities of everyday existence precluded taking the day off. For one thing, the early Christians did not come from the upper classes, at least not at first, and slaves and common people worked on Sunday. For another thing, the much-persecuted Christians were afraid to expose themselves by conspicuously not working when everyone else did.

Early in the second century, Pliny the Younger, the governor of a region in Anatolia (now Turkey), wrote a letter to the Roman emperor Trajan asking him what he should do about people who had been denounced as Christians. So far, he explained, he had interrogated each of them several times, and executed only those who refused to renounce their faith. But even that approach, tolerant as it was, made him queasy, because, he said, some of them had been guilty of little more than meeting before dawn on a "fixed day"—the assumption of many scholars is that the day was Sunday—where they would sing responsively a hymn to Christ "as if to a god," then "bind themselves by oath, not for any criminal purpose, but to abstain from theft, robbery, and adultery, to commit no breach of trust and not to deny a deposit when called upon to restore it." After that, they'd leave and assemble again later to eat—"food of an ordinary, harmless kind," Pliny added, as if to assure Trajan that the Christians were not eating the human flesh they were sometimes accused of sacrificing. And they had stopped holding even those meetings, Pliny said, "since my edict, issued on your instructions, which banned all political societies." (Worried that his prisoners may have lied to him, Pliny went on to clarify, he had tortured two female slaves known to their comrades as "deaconesses," but had not extracted from them any contradicting evidence.)

By the fourth century, however, everything had changed. In 321, the Roman emperor Constantine, the most important Christian convert in history, banned official business and manufacturing on Sunday; the day was clearly already holy to Christians throughout his empire. (Constantine exempted farmers, who urgently needed to bring their crops in, a move that shows how far Christianity had come from Judaism; Jewish Sabbath law specifically targets most forms of agricultural labor.) A decade earlier, on the eve of the battle in which he would conquer Rome and secure the title of emperor, Constantine granted his Christian soldiers Sunday leave so that they could worship in church, and required his pagan soldiers to recite a prayer on Sunday in which they praised the Supreme Deity without being forced to name him.

Constantine's knack for blending Christian faith and pagan syncretism was one of his great weapons as emperor. He became the first Christian ruler of Rome by sussing out points of convergence between paganism and Christianity. He took every opportunity to remind Romans that monotheism was not foreign to them, since they had already embraced monotheism—solar monotheism, the cult of Sol Invictus, the invincible sun. This deity, imported from the East in the middle of the third century and merged with the Greek figures Apollo and Helios, had become the chief object of the imperial religion. Before his conversion, Constantine had taken Sol Invictus as his divine patron; years after his conversion, his mints still struck coins featuring Sol Invictus as his patron. Constantine must have found it a most fortuitous coincidence that the Christians had settled on Sunday as the day of their Lord, since it was also the day set aside for worshipping the sun.

7.

IN ANTIOCH, a big, multicultural city in northern Syria, an up-and-coming preacher named John was also enraged by Sabbatizing. John would later come to be known as Chrysostom, or "golden mouthed," for the force of his oratory, and his attacks on the Sabbath would stick.

In a book titled *John Chrysostom and the Jews,* the historian Robert Wilken vividly reconstructs the scene. The year is 386 C.E. It is six decades since Constantine the Great converted to Christianity and declared Sunday a day of rest. Six years earlier, in 380 C.E., the Roman Empire declared Christianity its official religion. Christian Europe is in its infancy but has definitely been born.

Chrysostom, however, doesn't realize this. Christianity, to him, looks fragile, riven with squabbling and heresies and beset by enemies. In his youth, he lived through the brief reign of an anti-Christian emperor named Julian, who wrote a dyspeptic tract called "Against the Galileans." Chrysostom has no way of knowing whether this latest uptick in Christian-Roman relations will last. Paganism still shapes the public life of the Greek-speaking city. Its paintings, decorative mosaics, architecture, literature, and festivals all honor the glorious deeds of the Greek gods, not the redemptive powers of Jesus Christ. Antioch's ancient Jewish community also thrives. Though an anti-Jewish tone has crept into the language of Roman legislators whenever they address the rights of Jews in a Christian empire, few Jewish rights have actually been taken away, aside from the right to proselytize or to punish Jews who convert to Christianity.

In fact, the strength of Antioch's Jews alarms Chrysostom, since he finds himself competing with them for bodies in his church. The power of the Jews to lure away his congregants crests in the autumn, with the arrival of the Jewish High Holidays, when Jews prepare special foods, spruce up their homes, fast in repentance, build huts for Succoth, and dance in the public square—and many of their Christian neighbors abandon their churches to join them. "Many who belong to us and say that they believe in our teaching, attend their festivals, and even share in their celebrations and join in their fasts," Chrysostom thunders from the pulpit. "Many among us keep the Sabbath," he complains.

To keep Judaizers out of synagogue on Saturdays and Jewish holidays, Chrysostom employs some of the most violently anti-Jewish language used up to that point in Christian literature. His diatribes are a common form of preachment known as *Adversus Judaeos,* the sermon against the Jews, but Chrysostom embroiders his text with flowers of classical rhetoric, which teaches the art of slander as enthusiastically as the art of praise. Chrysostom's later readers will not recognize his strong words as typical Greco-Roman insults; his phrases will be taken literally, becoming a template for the anti-Jewish slanders that will follow in the centuries to come. Jews, he says, are dogs, gluttons, drunks, demons, thieves, cheaters, and child-murderers. They are wolves slavering over a soon-to-be-slaughtered Christian flock. Christians must do everything they can to keep them away: "Since today the Jews, more troublesome than any wolves, are about to encircle our sheep, it is necessary to arm ourselves for battle."

Wilken teases out a profile of the Judaizers who bother Chrysostom so much. They are neither recent converts from Judaism to Christianity nor old-time Jewish Christians. Rather, they are Christians from Chrysostom's own congregation who are drawn to Judaism by the very logic that drew them or their parents or grandparents to Christianity. Since God gave the Good Book to the Jews, and since they read it in Greek rather than in Hebrew, Jews must be closer to the truth than Christians. The Judaizers also admire piety. Chrysostom himself has to admit that the Jews care more about the Sabbath than his own flock does about Sunday:

> You Christians should be ashamed and embarrassed at the Jews who observe the Sabbath with such devotion and refrain from all commerce beginning with the evening of the Sabbath. When they see the sun hurrying to set in the west on Friday they call a halt to their business affairs and interrupt their selling. If a customer haggles with them over a purchase in the late afternoon, and offers a price after evening has come, the Jews refuse the offer because they are unwilling to accept any money.

The Judaizers see no reason not to go to synagogue on Saturday as well as church on Sunday. After all, Jesus kept the Sabbath and Passover. But Chrysostom knows that, inevitably, a Jewish festival will conflict with a Christian one, and that the ensuing squabbles will tear his church apart. If they keep the "fixed days" and "fixed times," Chrysostom tells his congregation, the Judaizers will "divide the assembly in two."

PART FIVE

PEOPLE OF THE BOOK

1.

I DIDN'T KNOW HOW TO PRAY. I STILL DON'T. THE TUNES, POURED INTO me as a child and dammed up through adulthood, spilled out with the tears, but the words had no meaning. If they possessed some sort of magic, I had no idea what it was. The prayer book, which must have had something in it to appeal to so many generations of Jews, had been turned by its translators into a gibber-jabber of exalted terms: rock, redeemer, raiments, majesty.

I also resisted the imperative to worship. Worship whom? Worship what? Wasn't that just mumbling and shuckling in the dark? The oppressiveness of the exercise was embodied in a phrase uttered just before an important prayer: "Open my mouth so that I may utter your praise." *Really?* I was to ask God to move my lips so that I could utter words that would gratify his ego? The sentence implied a closed robotic loop: I'd switch on God, and he'd operate my mouth by remote control.

What I liked was to walk to synagogue. In Park Slope, the route was a straight shot down Eighth Avenue. Nearly every house on the street was at least a century old, and all of them, if you looked at them long enough, seemed to stagger backward into history. They were drunk with weird period ornamentation. There was the Montauk Club, a Venetian palace ringed by terra-cotta heads of American Indians. There was the Adams House, half church, half castle, with heavy red Romanesque arches and a fairy-tale tower, built for the entrepreneur who invented both Chiclets and vending machines. There was Temple Beth Elohim, a 1920s synagogue with a surprisingly discreet presence on the street, given that its entrance, atop a sweeping staircase, featured Corinthian columns and grandiosely arched stained-glass windows, and behind those lay a pentagonal edifice meant to symbolize the five books of the Pentateuch.

At my synagogue, which lurked behind its dingy walls like an Eastern European *shtiebel,* I waited for the moment when they unrolled the Torah and chanted the sacred history, the chanters swaying over the pulpit like reeds in the wind. The light in which the patriarchs and matriarchs lived seemed brighter and cleaner—closer to Creation—than the brownish city light in which I moved. In it, contours sharpened; depths deepened. The men and women of the Bible were also spiritual superheroes, yet in their domestic lives they were mean-spirited, violent, pettily jealous. They spoke directly to God and dared to negotiate with him. Abraham bargained. Hagar begged. Rebecca complained. Moses placated. But they also coveted, lied, stole, murdered, raped. Jacob cheated Esau. Laban cheated Jacob. Jacob cheated him back. Jacob's sons murdered the inhabitants of a town who had agreed to convert to their faith, then sold their brother into slavery. Joseph, as a child, was an insufferable braggart.

But if the biblical personality possessed vitality rather than uplift, the biblical concept of time had a more palliative effect. Abraham was seventy-five when he left his home to follow God's call, and one hundred when Isaac was born. Isaac was forty when he married Rebecca. Jacob worked unhappily for his uncle for fourteen years. Women endured years without children, or hope of any. The success or failure of a biblical life was a thing to be determined in the epic mode, in the fullness of time between creation and redemption, not in an impatient New York season.

Enthralled as I was by the reading of the Torah, I was even more entranced by the ritual for taking it out of its cabinet, known, in a high archaism, as the Ark, after the box in which the Israelites carried it for forty years in the desert. It had been years since I went regularly to synagogue, and I had become enough of a stranger to see how odd this ritual was. You didn't just take out the Torah. You lifted it in your arms, cradled it, carried it around the room, kissed it, laid it down gently on the lectern, and blessed it over and over before you read it— chanted it, actually. Then you did the whole thing all over again before you put it away. This was idolatry of the highest order. The Torah might as well have been an infant Jesus, and we who carried it a procession of Madonnas. This wasn't just a religion of the Book. It was a fetish of it.

2.

WHENEVER PEOPLE BEGIN READING the Book, they start keeping the Sabbath. And when they keep the Sabbath they read the Book. It is no accident that religions centered on the Word of God and the texts in which it is written have set aside a day for absorbing them. If there hadn't been a Fourth Commandment, the people of the Book would have had to invent one. The ties that bind the Sabbath to the Book are also a closed loop. Driving it is the conviction—still held today, though as a highbrow rather than a devotional belief—that reading is a sacred act.

It was because they began to read Scripture—really to read it, every day, compulsively, in a desperate search for forgotten or obscured truths—that ordinary Christians experienced the lure of the Sabbath in the sixteenth century. And they began to read Scripture because, all of a sudden, they could. In 1517, when Martin Luther nailed to the door of a church in Wittenberg, Germany, a poster advertising a sermon in which he planned to advance ninety-five theses against the Catholic Church's trade in indulgences—forgiveness for sins, procured for a small sum—the printing press had existed for less than seventy years. (In Europe, anyway—new scholarship places its invention a generation earlier in Korea.) Printed matter was a novelty, though posters, pamphlets, and broadsheets had begun to sprout on city walls and street corners. Luther's attack on the Church may have been the spark that ignited the Protestant Reformation, but the kindling that caught and spread the fire was the fly sheets on which he had his theses printed and distributed throughout Germany. It took only two weeks for his views, which did not seem shocking to his fellow professors, to reach minds far removed from Wittenberg University and therefore less accustomed to sharp theological disputation.

Luther's outsized influence stemmed from his prescient grasp of the power of print. His Ninety-five Theses soon became a flood of tracts and pamphlets, written by him and by like-minded theologians and rebutted by their opponents. Luther wrote nearly as fast as the presses printed, supplementing his sermons and catechisms and broadsides with a new and soon-to-be-definitive translation of the Latin Bible into German. According to one estimate, one-third of all the books sold in Germany between 1518 and 1525 were written by Luther. "Printing," he declared, "is God's ultimate and greatest gift. Indeed through printing God wants the whole world, to the ends of the earth, to know the roots of true religion and wants to transmit it in every language. Printing is the last flicker of the flame which glows before the end of the world."

The marriage of print and religious polemic did not, in fact, herald the end of the world, but it did bring about something almost as revolutionary: "a truly mass readership and a popular literature within everybody's reach," in the words of the great French social historian Lucien Febvre. In Germany, literacy rates had doubled by the end of the century. Those who could not read found people to read to them. One study of a mining community in the Tyrol in the 1560s has groups of miners following a popular preacher from house to church to house on Sundays to hear him read from the Bible and preach out loud. In France, people reading forbidden books were prosecuted harshly, often by being burned at the stake. As a result, there are court records to tell us who they were: carpenters, barrel-makers, weavers, tailors, nail-makers, porters, pewter workers, leather workers, and furriers; respectable tradesmen as well as wandering journeymen; curates, students, schoolmasters, and doctors. And then there were the wives, sisters, and daughters of these men, some of whom were also burned at the stake.

To understand why reading became a mass phenomenon, you have to try to feel what these new readers felt. Religious reform, to them, was no remote technical matter. Attacking Church customs—indulgences, the saying of Masses for the dead, Latin liturgy, purgatory, celibacy, clerical immunity from civil taxes and laws, and traditional ceremonies and festivals—was a way of tackling the most pressing issues in any society in any era, which are: Who's in charge? Who gets to control the allocation of time and resources? What kind of regime should govern, and according to which code? Saying that the Church and its spokesmen should not dictate Christian practice and that individuals should determine their own devotional activities was to buck centuries of centralized authority. Luther's doctrine of *sola scriptura*—Scripture alone—reflected the fact that all religious laws that could be traced back to the Church and only to the Church had lost all legitimacy, at least in his eyes. If they were null and void, what code was there to follow but Scripture?

The Church had pushed the Bible so far to the margins of the religious experience that it wasn't even taught in most seminaries. Now people could read the Bible in their own vernacular languages, rather than struggle through it in Latin—and few had had the skills even to do that. Now they could interpret the text in the privacy of their homes and churches. And they could come up with their own original scriptural justifications for just about every aspect of life. Christ wouldn't have wanted things to be like this! That runs contrary to the Ten Commandments!

The consequences of translating the Bible, printing it, and putting it in everyone's hands cannot be overstated. People encountering God's word in their own languages felt, as if for the first time, pride in those languages, and in their own cultures. They were able to filter God's truths through familiar idioms, which made them more intimately their own. They could read the tale of nation-building in the

Old Testament and imagine themselves as part of a distinct nation, with its own destiny, rather than as, say, subjects of the Hapsburg or Holy Roman Empires. The Bible also raised for its readers questions of social organization. Hardly a political order dreamed up in the subsequent hundred years failed to have scriptural warrant behind it. By the seventeenth century, as the historian Fania Oz-Salzberger writes, "there were biblical royalists, biblical republicans, biblical regicides, biblical patriarchalists and defenders of the old order, biblical economic revolutionaries and deniers of private property, biblical French imperialists, biblical English patriots, and their biblical Scottish counterparts."

But no period was as radical as the first decade of the Reformation. Groups mushroomed overnight, joyously predicting the end of days. Iconoclastic mobs mauled statues of the Virgin Mary. Charismatic women cultivated followings, and, though women's thoughts had until then almost never found their way onto printing presses, these women went so far as to publish them. Evangelists renounced their clerical positions and moved to the countryside to preach a new social order to peasants. The ferment of the early Reformation came to a head in 1524, when uprisings swept across Europe in the massive upheaval called the Peasants' War. Inspired by the evangelists' preaching, peasants revolted against landlords, some of whom happened to be rich monasteries, and miners struck against kings. Princes and mayors and kings quashed the disturbances only through the application of extreme force, and rebels were slaughtered throughout the continent.

Luther was horrified, in part because he knew that his teachings shared some of the blame, and he and his fellow reformers promptly distanced themselves from the rebellion by aligning with the persecutory authorities—even with Catholic princes and monarchs—as they arrested and killed every religious radical they could find. But the excitement had spread and could not be quashed. Instead, it went underground.

It was at this point that the Reformation split in two. One half

cast its lot with the worldly authorities, advocated careful meliorist reforms, and eschewed anything that smacked too openly of anarchy or
heresy. This was the so-called Magisterial Reformation of Luther,
Huldrych Zwingli, and John Calvin. The other half, the Radical Reformation, was largely (though not entirely) made up of groups that
concluded that the quest for political power had been misguided and
withdrew from the world. This quietist attitude toward reform was
one part savvy and one part principle. Many of the founders of these
separatist sects had good reason to disappear, since they had helped
either to instigate or to fight the Peasants' War and were now being
arrested and executed. But some of them came up with a novel—and
very modern-sounding—argument for their quietism. They began to
promote what they called the Free Church. They argued that the
Church had grown corrupt when it acquired absolute power—when
Constantine converted and the papacy began and church married
state. If the Church were a true church of Christ, it had to be made
up of true believers, and "therefore could not be coterminous with
the physical boundaries of any one state or group of states," as historian Daniel Liechty puts it.

These proto-church-state separatists were called—by their enemies—Anabaptists, or re-baptizers, because they held that Christianity, being a voluntary faith, ought not to be forced on infants through
baptism. Only adults old enough to choose to join a Christian community were to be baptized; hence they rebaptized their first members, though later Anabaptists were baptized only when they came of
age, usually at thirty. (The Anabaptists of sixteenth-century Europe
were the direct precursors of the Anabaptists of twenty-first-century
America, that is to say, the Amish, the Mennonites, the Brethren, and
the Hutterites.) Two other groups to emerge during the Radical Reformation were the Socinians and the Unitarians. These eschewed
the doctrine of the Trinity—the creed that God was made up of the
Father, the Son, and the Holy Spirit—and some among them even
denied that Christ had been divine. Many in all of these sects were
pacifists; some were communists, believing that wealth should be

shared and property held in common; a few had female leaders. In manner of living, the Anabaptists and Unitarians were spare and ascetic. In style of worship, they strove to be biblical.

The key fact about the Radical Reformation, though, for our purposes anyway, was that when the sectarians read the Scriptures, they accepted no limits on their interpretive freedom. It was a common Reformation belief that Christianity had taken a wrong turn somewhere, usually with the papacy. All Protestants read Scripture for clues as to where and when that wrong turn came, no matter where this line of inquiry might lead. But the Anabaptists, appalled at the slaughter of the peasants, disgusted by Luther's support for it, alienated from Catholic and Protestant institutions alike, countenanced no check on the free play of their inquiries and refused to stop the search for a purer Christianity. Anabaptism spread most quickly among peasants and other people with little education, but its founders were learned men and original thinkers, and had become radicals in part because they had a passion for theological inquiry and were not afraid to cross the line into heresy. It was not long before someone came up with the notion that the fall of the Church should be traced all the way back to Christianity's break with Mosaic Law, and someone else traced it back to the abolition of the Saturday Sabbath.

Saturday Sabbatarianism made its first appearance, at least during the Reformation (scattered outbreaks of it had occurred before), in Silesia and Moravia—today parts of Poland and the Czech Republic—in the late 1520s, the innovation of two young intellectuals whose Anabaptist activities got them chased out of Germany and Austria. Oswald Glaidt was a former Franciscan monk and follower of Hans Hut, a millenarian who even after the slaughter of the peasants preached that the political authorities should be killed preparatory to the Second Coming of Christ. Andreas Fischer was less colorful but more systematic, and probably more influential. Together they formulated the theory and congregational practice of Saturday Sabbath worship. The Saturday Sabbath, they said, had been good enough for the patriarchs, as well as Moses, Jesus, and the apostles; therefore the Saturday Sabbath was good enough for all Christians. The Catholic

Church had upheld the command to refrain from work as moral, not ceremonial, and therefore binding on Christians, but decreed that the choice of day was ceremonial and therefore superseded, and that the Sabbath had mutated into the Lord's Day on the authority of the Church. Luther and Calvin also viewed the Fourth Commandment as only half binding, but since they refused to recognize the authority of the Church they considered one day to be as good as any other for resting (though Sunday would do fine). Luther said that although Sabbath rest was commanded, it should be wholly spiritual, not legalistic— that is, it ought not conform to rules and laws. Calvin denied that Sunday rest was commanded but considered it worth keeping because it was a social good, insofar as it promoted communal worship and general piety and gave servants a rest. Glaidt and Fischer, however, advanced the thesis that both parts of the Fourth Commandment—rest and Saturday observance—were moral and remained in force. The Sabbath, they said, would shed its rules and become purely spiritual only after Christ's resurrection.

It is hard for the modern mind to grasp how life-threatening such abstruse distinctions could be. When Luther learned what Glaidt and Fischer were preaching, he was furious. His reforms had already been tarnished by the Peasants' War. The last thing he wanted to hear was that Protestants had revived a ritual that reeked of Jewishness. In 1538, he wrote a treatise titled "Against the Sabbatarians" in which he called them "unlearned," "foolish" "apes," and "Judaizers." If they start keeping the Sabbath, he declared, the next thing they'll want is circumcision. (As Luther sputters and fumes his way through this essay, he mixes up the Judaizers with actual Jews. Early in his career, Luther had defended the freedom and dignity of Jews, whose refusal to convert he called a reasonable response to the nonsensical hash of Catholic doctrine; but when the Jews failed to convert upon hearing him, he decided they were hateful after all. "Against the Sabbatarians" is the first of many anti-Jewish works by Luther.) Calvin, for his part, said the Sabbatarians "went thrice as far as the Jews in the gross and carnal superstition of sabbatism."

Everything about the Sabbatarian Anabaptists seemed designed to outrage Luther in particular. Fischer, for instance, rejected Luther's distinction between Law and Gospel: "Christ did not come to abolish the Law but rather to give the believer power, through the Holy Spirit, to uphold it," as Liechty puts it. Fischer believed that what had led the church astray was its decision to replace the Jewish Sabbath with the Christian Sunday. Fischer, writes Liechty, "located the fall of the church exactly at the point where the church was cut off from its Judaic roots"; that was the moment, as far as Fischer was concerned, when the church stopped being the church."

About a year after Luther published "Against the Sabbatarians"— though not demonstrably as a result of it—Fischer was captured and killed by a Slovakian administrator loyal to the Hapsburg king of Austria, Ferdinand I, a Roman Catholic and harsh persecutor of Anabaptists. Five years later, Glaidt, who by then had probably abandoned his Sabbatarianism and joined a different Anabaptist group, the Hutterites, was taken to Vienna to be drowned in the Danube.

3.

INTELLECTUALLY, the Reformation was an exercise in nostalgia. Methodologically, it involved the rejection of texts from the recent Christian past—the abominations of the Church, as many reformers put it—in favor of texts dating back to a time when faith was believed to have been unperverted. Religiously, all this led back to Judaism. Reformation scholars (including Luther, at first) understood that if they were to cull lost meanings out of old books, they had to read them in the original, and if they were to disseminate those meanings, they had to retranslate the books and produce new commentaries that reflected their findings. To accomplish all this, they had to improve their Greek and Hebrew. Greek had enjoyed a revival during the Renaissance, but few Christian theologians in the early sixteenth century knew Hebrew. From whom would they learn it? From Jews and from Jewish sources, of course. Almost every serious Christian Hebraist found and cultivated a rabbi to be his instructor.

Modern scholars have only recently begun to appreciate the influence of Christian Hebraism on the Reformation. For one thing, until this century, few scholars of the period had the skills in Hebrew and rabbinics to understand it. For another, almost all sixteenth-century inquiries into Hebrew texts had the taint of controversy and were downplayed by later thinkers. Any Hebraist could be smeared at any time as a Judaizer, no matter how committed he was to Christian doctrine or how personally anti-Jewish (opposed to Judaism as a theological system) or anti-Semitic (opposed to Jews as a people). For this was still a time of expulsion, taxation, and ghettoization of Jews, when Jews still occasioned intense religious hatred and visceral social loathing. More pertinently, it was a time when Protestants felt vulnerable to the Catholic charge that they were backsliding into Judaism.

Worse, some Christian Hebraists went beyond learning Hebrew and began reading rabbinic writings, even borrowing from them. Scholars who felt they should be reading the Bible in its proper historical context, not through the filter of Christian supersessionism, looked to rabbinic texts for help interpreting biblical passages in light of their "plain," or historical, meanings, rather than their allegorical or typological meanings, that is, the way the verses were said to prefigure the Christ story. Other Christian Hebraists studied Kabbalah, or Jewish mysticism, in search of support for mystical Christian doctrines. But some Christian Hebraists who turned to rabbinic or mystical texts to elucidate Christian doctrine found that their studies did the opposite. They undermined core Christian tenets.

The best-known Christian Hebraic heretic was the sixteenth-century Spaniard Michael Servetus, who pointed out that mention of the Trinity could be found neither in the Bible nor in the writings of the early fathers. (It became doctrine at the Council of Nicaea in 325 C.E.) He made his point in a manner guaranteed to offend. Noting the absurdity of the claim that one is three and three is one, he declared, "Not only Mohammedans and Hebrews but the very beasts of the field would make fun of us if they could grasp our fantastical notion." Servetus exploited his knowledge of Hebrew to redefine the triune as three modes of *expressing* divinity, rather than *incarnating* it; he based this theological construct on the fact that the Old Testament uses several different names for God. The Catholic Church, Luther, and Calvin all recoiled at Servetus's gleeful and very Jewish-sounding debunking of the Trinity, which remained for them a mystery central to Christian faith. Servetus was burned twice—once in effigy by Catholics, the second time in the flesh by the officials of the city of Geneva, who had been pressed into action by Calvin.

Anabaptist Sabbatarianism had its fullest and longest-lasting flowering in Transylvania, where, not coincidentally, Servetus-style anti-Trinitarianism caught on with a vengeance. The rise, survival, and fall of the Transylvanian *Szombatosok* (Saturday people) is one of the most baroque episodes of sabbatizing in history, complete with freethinking religious intellectuals, Judaizing diplomats, court intrigues, harsh persecutions, forced conversions, secret rituals, and, finally, the Holocaust. Their story illustrates how the Hebraist logic led straight to Old Testament monotheism and biblical Judaism; it also affords a glimpse of that logic's appeal not just to elites but to common folk, whose Sabbatarianism probably had less to do with sympathy for the Jews than with the desire to defy their capricious and intolerant religious and political leaders.

Nowadays we think of Transylvania as a land dark with vampires and old castles, but in the late sixteenth century it was a country alive with ideas and unusually open to religious experimentation. Transylvania was a part of Hungary and the Hapsburg Empire, but by the sixteenth century, as a result of complicated politicking among Hapsburg princes, the Ottoman Empire, and Hungarian nobles, the region enjoyed the protection—though not the direct rule—of the Ottoman emperor Suleiman I, a man indifferent to the squabbles that had half of Europe trying to murder or excommunicate the other half. This put Transylvania beyond the reach of both the Church and the Magisterial Reformation. A highly diverse ethnic population also forced Transylvanians to cultivate the art of relatively peaceful coexistence.

Absence of censorship allowed the print industry to flourish and theologies to ramify. The Diet passed the first law in the West mandating religious toleration for different Christian denominations (Judaism and Islam remained forbidden). Lutheranism replaced Catholicism as the country's dominant religion, then was overtaken by the Calvinist Reformed Church. Francis David, the minister generally credited with founding Transylvanian Unitarianism, began as a Lutheran, became the leader of Transylvania's Calvinists, and then found himself questioning the Trinity. A debate was organized between David and the Calvinists.

It lasted ten days and has been called "the greatest debate in the entire history of Unitarianism." David argued the case for the doctrine of the Unity of God—that is, he maintained that the one God took precedence over the "persons" of God, a position that clearly threatened the divinity of Christ. By the ninth day everyone was tired and wanted to go home, so King John Sigismund of Transylvania adjourned the debate and called for another one. The second time around, David's opponent made so many nasty personal attacks on him that the king threatened to send the man home. In the end, King John sided with neither camp, but gave orders that the Unitarians not be interfered with. The Unitarians interpreted this as a victory and developed a rallying cry: *Egy as Isten,* "God is one!" By 1571, the king had converted to Unitarianism and passed a law recognizing the denomination as one of Transylvania's four religions, along with Lutheranism, Calvinism, and Catholicism.

But King John, the only Unitarian king in history, died early, by age thirty-one, and his Roman Catholic successor tamped down the country's religious freedom by adding a provision forbidding all religious innovation. David, meanwhile, had moved on from anti-Trinitarianism to non-adorantism, the refusal to address prayers to Jesus. He said that invoking Christ in prayers was no better than the popish practice of worshipping the Virgin Mary or dead saints. In 1578, so ill that he had to be carried into court, David was tried for the crime of innovation, condemned to life imprisonment, and died a few months later in a dungeon in a castle on a high hill.

Innovation was the charge, but the offense was Judaizing. Of that he may have been guilty, but less guilty than charged. In one of the stranger wrinkles in the plot, David was the victim of intellectual fraud. George Blandrata, an Italian Unitarian doctor who had fled persecution in Italy and become King John's physician as well as David's close friend and ally—he had, in fact, introduced David to Unitarian thought—decided David had gone too far and was endangering Unitarianism itself. Blandrata circulated a document in which David seemed to espouse the credos of a much more radical Christian Hebraist and anti-Trinitarian with messianic tendencies, Matthias Vehe-Glirius (his nickname was "the Jewish doctor"). This document claimed that Jesus spoke for God only insofar as his teachings conformed to the laws of Moses and the teachings of the Prophets. Though Jesus had preached a new covenant, it had not been accepted, and he had not freed his followers from the Law. Therefore the Old Testament should take precedence over the New until the Second Coming and Jesus' reign on earth.

Though this forgery led to David's death, it spread ideas among his followers that quickly blossomed into Sabbatarianism. Transylvania's first open Sabbatarian was a longtime friend and follower of David: Andreas Eossi, a nobleman who owned three villages and more estates and had lost three sons and a wife to illness. Old and sick, he comforted himself by reading the Bible, as well as the writings of Vehe-Glirius. "This man," wrote one seventeenth-century chronicler, "read the Bible so long that he extracted the Sabbatarian religion, with which he fooled a great many people." Eossi didn't just read; he wrote books, hymns, essays, and didactic poems. In them, he denied that Jesus freed his followers from the Law. One of the Church's many mistakes had been to abandon the Jewish calendar, and he founded a church that celebrated biblical festivals, especially Passover and the Sabbath. He called the Sabbath a "spiritual marriage" and welcomed it in wedding clothes. Eossi's ideas spread from village to village and ultimately reached the cities, becoming surprisingly popular among Transylvanian noblemen and noblewomen. By 1638, there were said to be between fifteen and twenty thousand Sabbatarians in Transylvania.

In 1583, a traveling Jesuit reported that a shocking number of Transylvanians "abstain[ed] from blood and pork," kept the Sabbath, ate unleavened bread, and practiced circumcision. In the 1590s, Tran-

sylvania came under the influence of a fiercely anti-Protestant emperor, Rudolf II, and in 1595 the Diet outlawed Sabbatarianism.
Some prominent Sabbatarians responded by sending a letter to the
military commander of the Turkish empire, pledging their loyalty to
the Turkish sultan. After that, their books were burned, their property
confiscated, their men flogged and jailed. In 1618, twenty-two Sabbatarian church buildings were seized and the Unitarians were forced
to expel the Sabbatarians from their church. Several Sabbatarians
went over to the Reformed Church.

They continued to keep the Sabbath in secret, though, led by
Simon Pechi, a diplomat whose life story sounds like something
dreamed up by John le Carré. He started out as Eossi's sons' tutor.
When Eossi's sons died, Eossi made Pechi his heir. Before that, however, he sent Pechi all over the world—Constantinople, North Africa,
Rome, Naples, Spain, Portugal. When Pechi returned, years later, he
spoke several languages and knew a surprising amount about rabbinic
Judaism. He married the daughter of a prominent Transylvanian family; became Transylvania's chancellor; negotiated a major peace ac-
cord in the Thirty Years War between the Turks and the Hapsburgs;
then fell from favor. The prince of Transylvania imprisoned him, took
away most of his property, and ended his career. This appears to have
reflected a change in the diplomatic climate, not anti-Sabbatarianism,
but his religious views couldn't have helped his cause.

The prince must have been fond of Pechi, though, because
shortly after jailing him, he allowed a group of Turkish Sephardic
Jews—descendants of the Jews expelled from Spain in 1492—to
move to Transylvania and granted them freedom of worship and
dress, rights denied them in most of Europe. After the prince died,
Pechi moved back to his one remaining estate and grew close to the
Jews, who had settled nearby. He set up a synagogue in his house,
translated portions of the Hebrew Bible and rabbinic literature into
Hungarian, wrote and compiled Sabbatarian hymns, and opened a
Sabbatarian school. Under Pechi, the Sabbatarians did not go so far as
to consider themselves Jews, but they did claim to be a foreign branch
grafted onto the Tree of Israel. They kept kosher and lit candles on

Friday nights. In 1639, during what has been called the Reformed Inquisition—an attempt to rid the country of radical Unitarianism—Pechi was condemned to death. He saved himself by converting to Calvinism.

Over the next few centuries, Transylvanian Sabbatarianism dwindled but did not disappear. It took root in a small village named Bozod-Ujfalu. Its adherents became an eccentric remnant of a forgotten schism, rather like the Amish in America. In 1855, one observer wrote:

> The thirty-eight Sabbatarian families (about 150 souls) outwardly belong for the most part to the Reformed Faith. Several, however, are Unitarians, only very few Greek-Catholics. On Sunday they visit the respective churches and listen with rapt attention whenever the clergymen recite quotations or narrative incidents from the Old Testament. On Christian festivals they keep away from church. On the Sabbath they hold divine service at home; but on the rest of their Jewish celebrations they meet in the house of a member which is devoted to the purposes of a synagogue, on which occasions Sabbatarians living elsewhere, especially those of Nagy-Ernye, attend. The service is conducted by one of the members, who is chosen rabbi, whom, however, they frequently change for another. Much superstition is mixed up with their belief. They can all read and write. They preserve their traditions faithfully, and boys of eight to ten years old can be heard talking about the history, adorned with legend, of Sabbatarianism and of Simon Pechi. Notwithstanding their communicativeness, they are very reserved as regards the books of their sect. They give their children for the most part Old Testament names, especially the name Moses. At marriages and burials they perform Jewish customs, before the Christian ones demanded by established religion take place. After marriage in church the Jewish marriage is solemnised. The women have their hair cut. A Sabbatarian girl never marries a Christian. Christian girls who would enter into matrimony with Sabbatarians must first pass a year of probation.

In 1869, two years after Hungary passed a law allowing Christians to convert to Judaism, its last handful of Christian Sabbatarians became Jews. During World War II, Hungary's pro-Nazi collaborators rounded up the Sabbatarians along with the rest of Transylvania's Jews and took them to a brick factory in a town near Bozod-Ujfalu. A local priest tried to rescue them by showing an SS officer forged baptismal certificates, but not all of them were willing to deny that they were Jews. Those who did not died in Auschwitz. It is said that after living in the brick factory for several days, the Sabbatarians and the other Jews of the region came to despise each other. The other Jews—few of whom still practiced their religion—refused to acknowledge the Sabbatarians as Jews, and the Sabbatarians replied that they were more Jewish than their accusers, because they kept the laws.

The Communists finally destroyed what the Christians and Nazis could not. In the 1980s, Nicolae Ceauşescu, the Communist dictator of Romania, decided to destroy more than seven thousand villages in Transylvania, which had reverted to Romanian rule after the war but whose inhabitants refused to consider themselves Romanians. In 1989, months before Ceauşescu and his wife were executed by firing squad, the Romanian army completed a dam and flooded Bozod-Ujfalu. After four hundred years, the Sabbatarian heresy was finally wiped out.

The *Szombatosok,* as it happens, was only one of many Anabaptist Sabbatarian groups, and not even the only one to survive into the twentieth century. Anabaptists kept the Sabbath on Saturday in Norway, Finland, Sweden, the Netherlands, France, Spain, and Russia, and were almost all persecuted for it. When a small sect of anti-Trinitarian Saturday Sabbatarians (Subbotniki) appeared in Russia in the early nineteenth century, probably under the influence of some Moravian Anabaptist refugees, the Russian government ordered that their leaders be drafted into the military for a lifetime of service or sent to Siberia and the rest be classified as a "Jewish sect." There are still Subbotniki in Russia today, most of them converted to Judaism, some of them seeking to make aliyah to Israel. In yet another of the dark historical ironies that have always seemed to characterize Sabbatarian history, rabbinic authorities in Israel empowered to determine who is a Jew have recently begun to challenge the validity of the Subbotniki's conversions and to refuse to grant them Israeli citizenship.

4.

ONE MORNING in synagogue, instead of listening to a sermon, we studied a passage in the Talmud about Hannah, the mother of the great judge Samuel. Before she gave birth to him, she had been another of the many biblical women driven to desperation by infertility. Where in the Bible, the Talmud asks, do we see true reverence—the biblical word means heaviness of head—in prayer? In Hannah, a rabbi named Elazar answers, when she begged God for a child. For "she was bitter of spirit," he says, quoting the Torah.

This was crazy! I knew Hannah's story very well, thank you, because Hannah was my Hebrew middle name, and once, as part of an assignment for a college fiction class, I had invented a character I named Hannah as a sort of alter ego. Then I had decided to read the story of the original Hannah. No one could be less of a paragon of rabbinic piety. Depressive and proud, prickly and dissatisfied, she tilted against everything in her life. Lacking children in a society in which a woman's worth was measured in children, she fought constantly with her husband's other wife, who had many sons and daughters and mocked Hannah for her barrenness. She wept and fasted and rejected her husband's efforts to comfort her, even though he openly preferred her to his other wife and, displaying an unusual degree of romantic love, at least for the time, asked her, "Am not I more to you than ten sons?"

Finally, during the family's yearly visit to a central shrine, she went to the sanctuary and prayed and wept with such soundless intensity that her lips moved but "her voice was not heard" and an elder priest had to rebuke her for praying while drunk. But then, rather than slink away ashamed, as one might expect a commoner to do after being reprimanded by a temple official, she boldly defended herself. "No, my lord," she said, "I am a woman of a sorrowful spirit: I have drunk neither wine nor strong drink, but have poured out my soul before the Lord. Count not thine handmaid for a daughter of Belial: for out of the abundance of my complaint and grief have I spoken hitherto." (The rabbis also thought her response bordered on arrogance. Pointing out that she started her reply with an unnecessary "No," they speculate that what she meant to say was—and I quote—"You do not know what you are talking about, and you must not be blessed with God's spirit, if you suspect me of such a thing.")

And here Hannah's story takes a surprising turn. For the priest does not take offense. Instead, he accepts her implicit reproach, draws himself up, and says, "Go in peace: and the God of Israel grant thee thy petition that thou hast asked of him." Shortly after that, she conceives Samuel, and once he is weaned she gives him to the priest to raise as a Nazirite, which is rather like giving him over to be raised by monks.

Hannah's voiceless despair, her deeply female alienation, her barely contained outburst at a priest—*this* exemplified prayerfulness? It seemed implausible that the rabbis, whom I thought of as villains of patriarchy, could have meant to advance such a protofeminist notion. And yet, it seemed, they did, or something like it. Our rabbi told us that tradition deemed Hannah the first Jew to engage in private prayer, as opposed to public ceremony. He pointed out Rav Hamnuna's wondering comment, "How many important laws" (Hamnuna meant about prayer) "can be learned from these verses relating to Hannah!" And our rabbi explained that there had been a reason to make her the exemplary figure of prayer. The silence that Eli mistook for inebriation gave the ancient rabbis the image of the sensibility they were trying to cultivate to replace the lost religion of priests and temple sacrifices. It was from Hannah that Jews were to learn *kavanah,* the rather Buddhist-sounding art of focusing one's soul inside oneself and burrowing deep into one's prayers.

This was, to me, a new idea. I had always thought of prayer as the repetition of ancient words praising a God I didn't believe in and

making promises I never intended to keep. As Heschel wrote somewhere, "Prayer is an extremely embarrassing phenomenon." If I concentrated hard enough, I thought, as I stared blankly at the prayer
book Saturday after Saturday in synagogue, maybe one day the words
would part like the Red Sea and their secret meanings would become
as clear to me as the sand on the floor of the sea.

In fact, it occurred to me, I was having such a moment right now.
A line from the Shemoneh Esrei popped into my mind, and I suddenly understood it. That was the prayer said silently, while standing,
which required the steps and bows I had not known in camp and still
didn't totally grasp. The petitioner praises God for "upholding the
fallen, healing the sick, freeing those in chains, and keeping faith with
those who sleep in the dust." And now I saw those lines through Hannah's eyes: God, I thought, is that which keeps faith with our desire to
believe that the bad—the intolerable—can improve, *must* improve,
which is part of the desire to believe in the intrinsic goodness of the
world. This is said to be the radical innovation of monotheism, for the
many gods in the pagan pantheons could not be counted on to further the interests of the common person. God was Hannah's conviction that she had the right to hope, despite having no reason to do so.
And prayer was her way of committing herself to that quixotic view.

I thought of my Hannah, who *was* a daughter of Belial. I had en-
visioned her as an artist's model living on the fringes of a big university, socializing with and seducing younger male students. Sarcastic,
lonely, a college dropout surrounded by future lawyers and doctors,
she knew that her boyfriends laughed at her even as they slept with
her, but she laughed back at them. Like the other Hannah, she held a
grudge against her body. It was not her ally; it did not help her find
her way in the world. She offered it up for casual sex and anatomical
studies destined to be absorbed into student art or discarded at the
end of the semester. And she nursed a grievance against everyone
who failed to register the depths of longing in her, even though she
could not have said what, exactly, she longed for.

The biblical Hannah, it occurred to me, was the principle of dignity my Hannah was trying to locate. The Hannah of old had in-vented not just inward prayer but inwardness itself—the psychologi-cal depth that comes from a ragged wound between inside and outside, between soul and body. Her anguished interiority meets with misunderstanding, but she has the resources to explain herself, to transform her outward identity from drunk or madwoman to symbol of piety.

As we talked about Hannah, my mind wandered to my mother, who, in the years since I had graduated from college and meandered around New York, trying to figure out what to do with myself, had figured out what to do with herself. She had moved to New York to go to graduate school, accompanied by my father, who sold his share in the family business and became a private investor. She had enrolled in a Ph.D. program at the Jewish Theological Seminary; switched to the rabbinical school in 1984, when the Conservative movement agreed to ordain women; and, at long last, making her childish fantasy an implausible reality, been ordained as a rabbi.

When she told me that she was going to rabbinical school, I had been as supportive as my self-image as a feminist required me to be, but inwardly I was horrified. Who would try to become a leader in a religion that did not consider you leadership material? I imagined my mother barging in where she was not wanted, making a spectacle of herself. Once, I got out of bed in the morning, went into her room, and found her wrapped in tefillin, the leather strips that Jewish men bind to their arms and heads during the morning prayers. I had never seen this done except at camp, and I had certainly never seen a woman do it. I backed out of the room quickly, unseen, as if I had just caught her cross-dressing. I got upset, too, every time I saw her up on the bimah, the platform in front of the congregation, reading Torah or leading prayers. She had had her bat mitzvah only a few years back. What if she made a mistake?

My mother graduated from rabbinical school in her fifties, and had not been offered a pulpit. The idea of a woman rabbi remained unthinkable to many congregations, and she had not been willing to leave New York to find a synagogue small enough or remote enough to be forced to hire one. Instead, she had become a hospital chaplain. My mother was an impatient woman, and had never had the knack of listening to other people talk about their pain, but she worked diligently at the task, and her supervisor praised her empathy and kindness. I ought to have been proud, but instead I was angry: She had turned into a glorified nurse, rather than a real rabbi! She was living proof that my skepticism about the possibilities for women in Judaism was warranted.

Nonetheless, I admired her more than I was willing to admit, and was jealous, too. She had graduated, Hannah-like, from silence to speech, which seemed more than I could say for myself. The more I thought about her, the more ashamed of myself I became, until I had to sneak out of the synagogue library and go calm down in the bathroom. When I got home, I decided it was time to quit messing around and call a psychoanalyst.

5.
——

ONE SATURDAY NIGHT in the fall of 1622, give or take a year, an eighteen-year-old student at Cambridge named Thomas Shepard got "dead drunke," as he later put it, and woke up the next morning in a place that he didn't recognize. He slunk away to a cornfield to sleep off the hangover. Shepard was in his third year at Emmanuel College and was destined to become one of the most beloved preachers in Puritan New England, as well as a founder of Harvard College. Shepard's magnum opus was *Theses Sabbaticae,* one of the great Sabbatarian tracts of the New World and the philosophical cornerstone of the American Sunday. (The Puritans never went so far as to embrace a seventh-day Sabbath.)

For the moment, however, he was just an undergraduate who kept fast company and liked to argue, he later explained, "about things which now I see I did not know at all but only prated about them." It's hard to imagine Thomas Shepard as an overconfident college student, because the literature that he left to posterity exudes self-abasement. His self-recrimination is no less convincing for having been obligatory, the practice of Puritanism having consisted in large part of sharp self-scrutiny in daily diary entries. He went out into the fields, he tells us, "in shame and confusion," and spent that Sabbath hiding in the corn, "where the Lord, who might justly have cut me off in the midst of my sin, did meet me with much sadness of heart and troubled my soul for this and other my sins."

Shepard was born in 1605 in Towcester, a small town in the English Midlands. He was the son of a grocer's apprentice and a grocer's daughter. His mother died when he was four. His father remarried, but his new wife disliked Thomas and turned his father against him. Soon afterward, he was sent to a school run by a "curst and cruel" headmaster, who made him wish that he could keep "hogs or beasts rather than go to school and learn." His father died when he was ten, and his stepmother refused to spend the £100 allotted to her for his education. Eventually he was rescued by an elder brother and a friendly local preacher and became a passionate scholar. But he never quite managed to convince himself that he hadn't somehow brought his unhappy childhood on himself, perhaps, he conjectured, by his own irremediable "childishness." He considered it his mission in life always to keep before his mind his own "vileness."

At the age of eighteen, though Shepard didn't know it yet, he was embarking on his conversion. This, another Puritan rite of passage, nonetheless had in his hands the ring of genuine anguish. The hurdle to be overcome was a deep ambivalence toward all things religious. "I questioned whether there were a God," he wrote, "whether Christ was the Messiah, whether the Scriptures were God's word or no. I felt all manner of temptations to all kinds of religions." Was his faith just a product of his education? Had he been raised Catholic, would he have thought that popery was the truth? And if that were true, did it not mean that his faith could just as easily be false as true?

What rescued him from his apostasy and brought him to redemption? Shepard never comes out and says so, but the close reader of his autobiography would have to say that it was the Sabbath. It was on Sundays that, inspired by the kindly preacher, he began to educate himself by taking notes on the sermons. Ignorant and undisciplined, he wasn't able to take the notes at first, but then he prayed, and lo and behold, the following Sunday he succeeded. After years of godless scholarship at Cambridge, he began to go on Sunday to hear the sermons of the master of Emmanuel, which allowed him to experience the terror of God's wrath. The drinking binge occurred on a Saturday night, and he came to on a Sunday. That was when a fearful intuition of God's presence began "to break in like floods of fire into my soul," he wrote, until he had "some strong temptations to run my head against walls and brain and kill myself."

Finally, "on a Sabbath day at evening," it occurred to him to "do as Christ"; that is, when Christ was in agony, he fell to his knees and prayed. Whereupon God filled him with his spirit, allowing him to grasp the depths of his unworthiness. Years later, in the *Theses Sabbaticae*, Shepard wrote that "religion is just as the Sabbath is, and decays and grows as the Sabbath is esteemed: the immediate honor and worship of God . . . is nursed and suckled in the bosom of the Sabbath."

A decade after Shepard's conversion, the Anglican archbishop of Canterbury, William Laud, began to persecute Puritan ministers for nonconformity. Laud, embittered by the harsh Puritan critique of his Church of England and weary of fending off accusations that Anglicans were depraved because they allowed dancing and gaming on Sunday afternoons, decided to remove Puritans from English churches. Shepard was among the many whom he called to his chambers and forbade to practice as a minister. Shepard spent four years preaching on the sly, chased around England by Laud's officers, and finally set out for New England. He and his wife and son had sailed only a few miles when they were driven back to shore by a sudden storm. True to the pattern, they nearly foundered on rocks on a Saturday and were rescued on a Sunday. Shepard felt that they had disembarked prematurely. They should have stayed on board and sung their grateful Sabbath hymns.

6.

THE PURITAN SUNDAY, the historian M. M. Knappen wrote, represents "a bit of English originality." That's a wry way of describing an institution that defies comprehension by anyone not a Puritan. To the modern mind, the desire to strip the day of all lightheartedness and pleasure—of piping and minstrelsy, wakes and feasts, plays and the frequenting of alehouses, to name a few of the Sunday activities targeted by Puritan legislators in the seventeenth century—can be explained only as the war of a joyless bourgeoisie against a subversively festive peasantry.

That was the Marxist historian Christopher Hill's take on English Sabbatarianism, anyway. To understand the Puritan approach to the Sabbath, he thought, you had to know that Protestants throughout Europe strove to do away with the more than one hundred saints' days observed by the Catholic Church every year. The Puritans also banished Christmas and Easter. Among other things, Hill said, these holidays interrupted what were felt to be the proper rhythms of labor. As England industrialized, regular work habits and synchronized schedules became the keys to success. Popery, Slingsby Bethel wrote in 1668, drove "the industrious sort of people" into hiding. The Sabbath, on the other hand, came around predictably. Moreover, the Fourth Commandment explicitly states that on six days of the week you shall work. The Puritans were committed to rooting out idleness, "the mother and breeder of vagabonds," in the words of one Robert Hitchcock.

The Sabbath also gave these proto-workaholics a way to escape their own hypertrophied work ethic. Sunday Sabbatarianism could be seen as an early form of labor consciousness. The Industrial Revolution was in its infancy, but the old guilds were dying, and in many new industries there were no guilds at all. Competition was cutthroat. The small producer or businessman felt driven to work long hours, seven days a week, and to make his apprentices and journeymen do so as well. The only way to protect the "industrious sort" from themselves, Hill wrote, was to prohibit Sunday work and travel, and to enforce this prohibition strictly. Who had the authority to enact and enforce such prohibitions? Not private citizens and not guilds, but church-wardens backed by local magistrates.

Another explanation for the Puritan Sabbath is social-psychological. In his *Revolution of the Saints* (1965), the political philosopher Michael Walzer explains the Puritan fanaticism for order as not just a political response—the answer to industrialism—but a gut feeling of insecurity. England in the seventeenth century was a country racked by change. The population exploded at the very moment when the countryside became unlivable for many, owing to something called "enclosure"—the fencing off of communal lands into private plots, most of them owned by manorial lords. Beggars took to the roads and jammed the cities. Thomas Hobbes wrote menacingly of "masterless men." The cities' suburbs and outparishes housed the displaced throngs. The old Church had collapsed, as well as the guilds, and with them many of the civic institutions that linked people to one another. "How were men to be reorganized, bound together in social groups, united for cooperative activity and emotional sustenance?" Walzer asks. "Deprived of village solidarity, disoriented in the great crowds, many men must have found solace in Puritan faith." The Puritan an-swer to social disorder was the congregation, or the "good company," a community in which godliness and orderliness were the rule. When did that congregation unite into a community? When it gathered on Sunday, of course.

But another way to think about the Puritan Sunday is that it served as a doorway into something the Puritans held dearer than just about anything else: the Bible, the revelation of the Word and Will of God. Puritanism can be seen as a glorious, centuries-long exercise in biblical reenactment. Imagine the Civil War reenactments that occa-sion such religious adherence in our time, and then imagine them as an actual religious movement. Puritanism, in historian Theodore Dwight Bozeman's memorable formulation, was a form of "Biblical primitivism."

That is, admittedly, putting matters a little starkly. For one thing, the Puritan Sabbath was the product of a very complex and contemporary evolutionary process, not a simple reconstruction of the biblical Sabbath. Insofar as the Puritan Sabbath had been shaped by English Sabbatarianism, it was not even, strictly speaking, Puritan. What we think of as the English Sabbath antedated by decades the advent of what we call Puritanism. (Puritans did not call themselves by that name; they were called that by those who objected to their efforts to "purify" the Church of England.) In the seventeenth century, however, during the Puritan ascendancy in England and among the Puritan Separatists who moved to America, Sabbatarianism attained a degree of importance never seen before or after in Christian history.

John Hooper, a bishop of England and Worcester under King Edward VI who had lived in exile in Protestant Zurich during the reign of Henry VIII and was martyred under the reign of the Catholic Queen Mary, fleshed out the rudiments of the theology of the English Sabbath in 1558.

There are four main points of English Sabbatarian theology. First, the Sabbath was to be kept on Sunday, not on Saturday—though it was stressed that the day had been transferred from Saturday to Sunday by biblical authority, not at the whim of the Church. According to Hooper, when Paul called for Christians to give alms to the poor on Sunday in First Corinthians, he made Sunday the Sabbath. (Saturday Sabbatarianism does make the occasional appearance in Puritan thought, but these inklings were dismissed as Judaizing and yielded churches only in the seventeenth century, with the advent of the Seventh-Day Men and the Baptist movement.)

Second, the Fourth Commandment is moral, therefore still binding; its only ceremonial aspect is the injunction to keep the Sabbath on the seventh day, a time that was deemed more suitable to Israelites than to Puritans. The word *moral* may be too mild to convey the enormity of the goodness that the Sabbatarians ascribed to the Sabbath. For the Puritans in particular, the morality of the Sabbath lay in its being rooted in the nature of things, part of the law that God embedded in the universe at Creation. One theologian, Richard Greenham, went so far as to claim that the Fourth Commandment was the only one given to Adam and Eve in the Garden of Eden. In *Theses Sabbaticae,* Shepard explained that God's "moral law," the Ten Commandments, was written first upon the heart of man in "his primitive and perfect estate." After mankind's fall, however, God had it written down in stone.

Third, the Sabbath is a social and personal discipline. It is a means—for the Puritans, the chief means—of sustaining the order and holiness of a sanctified life. The Puritan Sabbath included a vigorous menu of spiritual exercises. It entailed extensive preparation beforehand; the good Christian was to quit work at midday on Saturday to get himself and his family and his servants ready for the Sabbath, and to predispose their hearts for grace. This labor included, among other things, conducting a tally of sins committed during the week, and repenting for them. The day itself involved public worship, reflection and study, and acts of mercy or charity toward the poor. The goal of all these Sabbath activities was to achieve a prelapsarian purity, "to bring ourselves back into that estate, from whence we are fallen, and as it were to recover our first footing," wrote Nicholas Bownde in *The Doctrine of the Sabbath* (1595).

Fourth, however, and most important for a Puritan, the Sabbath was the only day on which ordinary people could fully bask in the glory of the Word. For at the heart of the Puritan quest for grace lay a search for the Word, uncorrupted and unmediated and free of High Anglican rhetorical flourishes, and Sunday was the day of the Word's dominion. It was preached in sermons—Puritanism's highest literary form—sung in psalms, read in Scripture, meditated upon in private, and discussed in public in appropriately godly conversations.

Though the Word was to be kept plain, its dissemination did not lack for theatricality. Puritan preachers roamed the English countryside, teaching the Bible to anyone who would listen and cultivating an aura of rustic simplicity. According to the historian William Haller, who draws his observations from the work of the seventeenth-century Puritan biographer Samuel Clarke, anyone who met the minister John Carter and his wife, for instance, "would say, they had seen Adam and Eve, or some of the old Patriarchs." Haller continues, evocatively: "They lived and dressed as plain as Jacob and Sarah, and had only utensils of wood, earth, pewter, and brass, no plate. The wooden salt-dish had grown black with age and use. The 'house was a little Church.' Thrice a day the scriptures were read and the children and servants catechized and instructed. All comers were welcome. There was always a 'wholesome, full, and liberal diet . . . and all fared alike: He and his wife did never think that his children and servants and poor folk did eat enough.' " It was a merry saying among the godly that "if they would be a Cow or a Horse or a Hog or a Dog, they would choose Master Carter for their master."

Puritanism was as much a style as a theology, and it is in its style that we can discern its leveling nostalgia, its urge to wipe away the distortions of human history. The Puritans would have said they were fleeing the present time of weakness for a Great or Strong Time. David D. Hall, a cultural historian, calls the Puritan style "the new protestant vernacular." He describes the fashions in vogue among the settlers of New England: "Psalm-singing replaced ballads. Ritual was reorganized around the celebration of the Sabbath and of fast days. No town in New England had a maypole; no group celebrated Christmas or St. Valentine's day, or staged a prelenten carnival. New England almanacs used numbers for each month instead of names deemed 'pagan.' " When parents named their children, they chose biblical names: John, Joseph, Samuel, James, and Timothy for boys and Mary, Elizabeth, Sarah, Hannah, Abigail, Rebecca, and Ruth for girls.

The Puritan Sabbath, for the pious Puritan, did not consist of long, throttling hours of enforced inactivity. Underneath its carefully choreographed plainness, the day crackled with high drama and sensual joy. It's just that all these things happened inside the soul, not out in the world. Sinners entered the presence of God on this day of "state and royal majesty, when all his saints compass his throne and presence," Shepard wrote, and repent the "soil" and "decays" of the week before. And they were to lie with Jesus, "in the bosom of his sweet mercy," the whole day long, and he would rest with them, tenderly, lingeringly.

Puritans disapproved of the theater as a cultural institution because it distracted from the greater drama of the struggle for redemption. But nonetheless, on the Puritan Sabbath, mimetic rules applied. It was necessary to follow the letter of the law, in part because God commanded it but also in order to re-create the requisite atmosphere. Shepard called for the New England Sabbath to begin at sundown, as it does in the Old Testament. At that point, all work was to stop. He made use of traditional Christian definitions of work, distinguishing between servile works—labor done for worldly gain, profit, or livelihood, in order to acquire and purchase the things of this life—and works of preservation that made life tolerably comfortable. There was to be no "buying, selling, soweing, reaping"; nothing that could be done the following day, including bringing in the harvest or setting sail or cleaning house. But one was permitted "to rub the ears of corn, to dress meat for the comfortable nourishment of man," or "to pull a sheep out of a ditch, to quench fire in a town, to save corn and hay from the sudden inundation of water, to keep fire in the iron mills, to sit at stern and guide the ship."

All this not working and not playing certainly made the day quiet. "Sweet to the Pilgrims and their descendants was the hush of their calm Saturday night, and their still, tranquil Sabbath—sign and token to them, not only of the weekly rest ordained in the creation, but of the eternal rest to come," Alice Morse Earle wrote in a nineteenth-century paean to the early New England Sabbath. "No work, no play, no idle strolling was known; no sign of human life or motion was seen except the necessary care of patient cattle and other dumb beasts, the orderly and quiet going to and from the meeting, and at the morning, a visit to the churchyard to stand by the side of the silent dead."

Biblically inspired though it may have been, the Puritan Sabbath had a rigor all its own, particularly in New England. On Saturday night, the pious New England Puritan would gather the members of his family and household together and catechize them. On Sunday they went to the meeting house, called there at 9 A.M. by the blowing of horns or conch shells or the beating of drums. There they sat through two services, one in the morning and one in the afternoon, with a break in the middle of the day for lunch. Sermons were known to last for as long as four turnings of the hourglass. The Puritans chose not to heat their meeting houses, nor did they build backs on their pews. Some women brought coal foot stoves in the wintertime, and some towns had a noon-house, a low, stablelike building nearby, in which they built a fire, and where people who came from far away could eat and rest and warm themselves. Should a churchgoer nod off to sleep, he might be woken by a tithing man, a member of the congregation appointed to wander the building with a long staff. The staff had a knob on one end and a foxtail hanging from the other, and the tithing man would either rap the sleeper on the head or slap the fur against her face until she woke up.

How else would the Puritans have enforced such demanding religious discipline? The first Puritan colony in Massachusetts had no written code of laws; it was governed by magistrates interpreting the Word of God. But, by 1635, several Puritan ministers had begun to draft some. The very first code of laws—never actually adopted—was called Moses' Judicials, and it pursued the long-cherished aim of creating a holy commonwealth. Citing the tale of the wood gatherer in Numbers, who was put to death for violating the Sabbath, Moses' Judicials called for capital punishment for Sabbath-breaking. Later, Thomas Shepard was drafted to help write more reasonable laws, and in 1648 the General Court published *The Book of General Laws and Liberties.*

These were the blue laws, so called either because of the blue paper on which an early history of Connecticut was written and in which the laws were outlined, or, more likely, because *blue* meant rigidly moral in eighteenth-century slang. The laws made Sabbath church attendance compulsory; outlawed the denial of the morality of the Sabbath; prohibited Sabbath-breaking; and strictly punished acts of Sabbath burglary, which was rampant, given that houses often stood unattended all day long while their owners went to church. Other states soon followed Massachusetts' lead.

Enforcement of these rules was never quite as draconian as one might think from the horror stories promulgated even at the time. It is doubtful, for instance, that a man was ever actually put in the stocks for kissing his wife on the Sabbath. The court's most common response to Sabbath-breaking was admonishment. On the other hand, people were flogged, branded, put in stocks, and made to pay steep fines for breaking the Sabbath. The harshest punishments were for Sabbath burglary and other crimes committed on the Sabbath. But even if the actual penalties didn't always meet the standard of severity called for in the law books, the matter did not lack for attention. The court records brim with arrests, fines, and admonishments for everything from catching eels on Sunday and riding too "violently" to wringing out one's laundry and sitting under the apple tree with one's beloved. Walking, traveling, or visiting on the Sabbath could result in a fine. Failing to go to church almost certainly would.

A decade later, thanks in part to these laws, the Sabbath had become an entrenched American institution, kept even in towns filled with converted Indians. Though the actual number of American Puritans was never large, the Puritan Sabbath—enshrined in law by vigorous, literate leaders and bolstered by the Sabbatarianism that held sway in England in the seventeenth century—dominated the American Sunday until the beginning of the nineteenth century, at least in the northern half of the country. (Puritanism never found a foothold in the South.) Nonetheless, as soon as the Puritans passed their Sunday laws, and even before they did, the courts found themselves embroiled in battles over civil and religious liberty. The dissenter Roger Williams began his long career of annoying Bay Colony leaders by opposing their right to punish Sabbath-breakers. He was later exiled from Massachusetts and went on to found the colony of Rhode Island, the first to enshrine in law freedom of conscience and separation of church and state. A powerful splinter group called the Antinomians, led by Anne Hutchinson, derided laws enforcing Sabbath worship and behavior as "legalistic." A wave of Quakers came to New England in the late 1650s and fell afoul of the Sabbath laws by refusing to appear at Sunday public-worship services and holding their own meetings instead.

The Sabbath laws were among the most divisive of Puritan policies, and may well have provided the most ammunition, over the centuries, for the enemies of Puritanism. By the nineteenth century the Sabbath laws were a symbol of the Puritans' indifference to, and even intolerance for, individual pleasures and religious freedoms, as well as their will to compel worship rather than allow it to emerge from natural feelings. The laws were so controversial, even as they were being written, that you have to wonder what blinded the Puritan fathers to the inevitable repercussions. Why did they not worry about backlash? What was in their minds?

They were thinking of the Bible, of course. It stood before them as the text of reality, more real than life itself. It was not just *a* but *the only possible* model of society. Consider the biblical terms that Thomas Shepard uses when he justifies the use of state power to enforce a narrow notion of Sabbath rest. "Children, servants, strangers who are within our gates," he wrote, in a direct echo of the Fourth Commandment, "are apt to profane the Sabbath; we are therefore to improve our power over them for God, in restraining them from sin, and in constraining them (as far as we can) to the holy observance of the rest of the Sabbath." And if parents must keep their children from breaking the Sabbath, then how much more must the state keep its citizens from doing the same? Puritan political theory was nothing if not patriarchal. As Shepard wrote, invoking Nehemiah: "And if superiors in families are to see their gates preserved unspotted from such provoking evils, can any thing be but that the same bond lies upon superiors in commonwealths, who are the fathers of these great families, whose subjects also are within their gates, and the power of their jurisdiction?"

Historical hindsight makes it all too easy for us to see why some people might be oblivious to the larger blessings of the day. For one thing, the Puritan Sabbath had its morbid side. To be a Puritan was to live in a perpetual state of unfulfilled and unfulfillable expectation, for to the Calvinist death was certain, but redemption could never be. The Puritan Sabbath, like the Puritan diaries, was a tool of anxiety management. It allowed the Puritan to master his fear of the passage of time, and of death. You died for a day, and if you did it right, you got a taste of eternal rest. You prepared for the Sabbath as you prepared for heaven, Shepard said in the *Theses Sabbaticae*.

For the orphan from Towcester, however, the Sabbath offered respite from the harsh anguish of self-doubt. Sunday was the day when you made time for God, but also the day when God—that overworked parent—made time for you. A person like Shepard, who considered himself fit "to be forever banished from the presence of the Most High," and "exceedingly unworthy to come into it," could not fail to prize "this day to come and enter into [Christ's] rest, and lie in his very bosom all the day long, and as a most loving friend loth to part with them till needs must and that the day is done."

7.

No matter how much the Transylvanians and the Subbotniki suffered, or how long and hard the Puritans struggled, for their Sabbaths, their Sabbatarian obsessiveness could not match that of the Kabbalists, whose mystical theology predated and, through the Christian Hebraists, may have influenced the Reformation and came to a head in the sixteenth century. "It would be no exaggeration to call the Sabbath *the* day of the Kabbalah," wrote Gershom Scholem, the twentieth-century scholar of Kabbalah. These mystics kept the Sabbath not because they were commanded to but because that was how they made sure the world continued to exist.

It was the virtue of the Kabbalists to take the rituals and texts of biblical and rabbinic Judaism and imbue them with new meanings and an almost unlimited power to affect the world. The two most appealing features of mysticism are that it turns decayed metaphors into vibrant cosmic realities, as if letting a primordial poetry loose upon the world; and that it endows the mystic with uncanny powers. The mystical sense of agency—religious scholars call it theurgy, the notion that human actions can compel parallel actions in the divine sphere—dispels the impotence felt by the pious person when confronted with the presence of evil in God's universe. In the Kabbalistic system, the most mundane feat of ritual observance echoed in the heavens, and had the capacity to ensure the ongoing goodness of Creation. Mysticism turns the God of rationalistic theologies from someone you study into someone you experience directly. So when a Kabbalist kept the Sabbath he—and it was mostly, though not entirely, men who actively kept the Sabbath—didn't just *remember* Creation. He *renewed* Creation. He didn't just align himself with God's calendar; he sustained its very existence. When he rested, he didn't just imitate God; he helped God heal a broken world.

Kabbalists wove every ritual, no matter how trivial, into the plot of a cosmological drama. Consider the Sabbath preparation outlined by the historian Elliot Ginsburg, who, in an impressive feat of scholarship, has gathered together everything that is known about the Kabbalistic Sabbath. Rabbinic Judaism always required that one's house be made ready for the Sabbath, but the Kabbalists, with typical intensification, required you to sweep out cobwebs, as if evil itself lurked in the bodies of spiders. You festooned the house and the dinner table with pillows and embroidered cloths, as if welcoming a bride to a wedding—to a wedding canopy, or chuppah, to be exact. (Another common image is that of the bridal bedchamber.) For on the Sabbath, according to the great Kabbalistic texts, the female and the male aspects of God met and married. The Shekhinah, or Presence, of God, as she was called in the myth system of the Kabbalah, became one with her lover, Yesod (that is, the heavenly phallus) or with Tiferet, the principle of divine activity or the axis of the world—in short, with God's male emanation, whatever his name.

To take another example of mystical intensification, Kabbalists turned the usual Friday bath into an act of radical spiritual transformation. According to Moshe de Leon, the author of a classic thirteenth-century Kabbalistic text called the Zohar, a Jew bathes before the Sabbath to get away from the "other," or evil, spirit that rules during the week, and enters into "the other, holy spirit," in order that "he might receive the supernal holy Spirit." This is the Sabbath soul, the *neshama yeterah*. De Leon thought that this soul supplemented and strengthened the weekday soul. Later Kabbalists said that the Sabbath soul killed off the mundane soul every week in order to allow the Sabbath one to enter. Isaac Luria, the great Kabbalist from the northern Palestinian town of Safed, a center of Kabbalistic thought and activity in the seventeenth century, was said to be able to detect which soul was occupying a mystical adept on the Sabbath by studying that adept's forehead. Hayyim Vital, one of Luria's disciples, tells us that Luria once spotted the soul of the great biblical king Hezekiah on Vital's forehead. Later that same Sabbath, however, Vital had a temper tantrum, whereupon the soul of Hezekiah fled.

Kabbalistic Sabbath preparation spared no part of one's house or person. My favorite rule is one instructing the adept to pare the nails. De Leon hallowed fingernails and toenails above other parts of the body, for, he said, they are all that remain of a primordial garment worn by Adam in the Garden of Eden before the Fall, sometimes called a "chariot of light." Nails, de Leon said, mark the border between the sacred and the mundane, and that border must be purged of all filth before the Sabbath. And not only that; the nail clippings must be disposed of properly, as befits sacred refuse: "Three things were said in reference to nails: One who burns them is pious, one who buries them is just, and one who throws them away is a villain," as one Talmudic saying has it. This was the Kabbalist's standard procedure, to seize upon a chance Talmudic remark and embroider it until a new ritual emerged, rich with esoteric backstory. According to Lawrence Fine, Luria's biographer, Luria took a hint from the mention of a rabbi from the Talmudic era who stood at sunset to greet the Sabbath Queen, and developed a Sabbath dramaturgy that still has a powerful appeal to the modern sensibility and is echoed in today's Friday-night liturgy. On Friday nights, he and his followers went out to the fields outside Safed—to the "field of holy apple trees," trees being a symbol of the masculine aspect of God—to welcome the Sabbath bride. Dressed in white—for "the color of the garment one will wear in the world to come, following death, will be the same color as the clothes we wear on the Sabbath in this world"—they faced west, holding their hands in particular positions on their breasts that echoed the placement of cosmic forces in the universe.

When they went home, they circled their tables with myrtle in their hands, myrtle having been used once upon a time to make bridegrooms' wreaths, and also as an allusion to a story in the Talmud about a man who held two bundles of myrtle in his hand on the Sabbath, one to "remember" and one to "observe." They had their wives bake twelve loaves of challah, instead of the usual two, and place them upon the table, since twelve showbreads had been laid out in the Temple on the Sabbath. And they had sex with their wives every Friday night, whenever the women were not menstruating, in compliance with a detailed script. Luria, who seems to have been rather obsessive-compulsive, specified the time (after midnight), conditions (total darkness), and position (head facing east, feet facing west, right hand south, left hand north). Happily for the wives, the Kabbalist was also supposed to arouse his wife's desire before initiating sex. For these sexual activities, too, had God-changing implications. Sabbath orgasms echoed in the highest spheres of the sky, where the masculine and the feminine aspects of the Godhead were also trying to achieve their requisite Sabbath coupling.

Anyone watching these proceedings who was not familiar with their mythological depths would surely have thought himself in the company of madmen, but I can't help envying the Kabbalists. They found a way to overcome the alienation that chills our sensation of holy—its way of reminding us how far from God we really are. They felt themselves to be not just part of an intentional community but to dwell at the very center of the cosmos, which hung on their every act. "If the whole universe is an enormous complicated machine," Gershom Scholem wrote, "then man is the machinist who keeps the wheels going by applying a few drops of oil here and there, and at the right time."

8.

READING THE TALMUD ONE DAY, I came across the phrase *tinok she-nishba,* "the child who was captured." The rabbis were discussing the legal implications of forgetting the Sabbath—not just forgetting that it happens to be Saturday, so that you inadvertently perform a *melachah,* but forgetting, or perhaps not even knowing, that such a thing as the Sabbath exists. What would the penalty for such amnesia or ignorance be? Should there be one? And what kind of Jew could be so oblivious to the Sabbath? Only, the rabbis thought, a Jew who had suffered extreme cultural dislocation. Only a Jew who had been kidnapped as a child and raised by non-Jews.

Tinok shenishba turns out be a technical category in Jewish law, one that gets thrown in the faces of secular Jews—Jews who are ignorant of, or oblivious to, the rules. Had I known that at the time, I might have been insulted. Luckily, I didn't, so I seized on the romantic image and let it take me to all sorts of fanciful picture-postcard locales, gleaned from random book reviews: the Palestinian desert; the Italian ghetto, where Catholic nannies kidnapped their Jewish charges; Latin America, land of Marranos.

Raised by well-intentioned Jews, taken to synagogue on Sabbaths and holidays, given a bat mitzvah, currently residing in New York, the most Jewish city outside Israel, by what excess of self-pity could I possibly claim affinity with Jews like that? By what enemy had I been captured? By the enemy, I thought, that is myself. By my disdainful teenage self, which sneered at the cheap brutalist architecture of the suburban synagogue that we joined when we left San Juan for Miami, as well as at the windowless sanctuary filled with old women in hats. By my willful, authority-baiting self, which smoked dope behind my after-school Hebrew school, before and after class. By my cynical self, which scoffed at my parents' Holocaust obsession and the endless pictures of dead Jews in their library. By my lit-crit self, which read the world against itself. By my grandiose, ambitious, jealous self. By every self that I had been and seemed destined to become. I wanted to be reborn, fresh and pure. I wanted to be led back to the paths of righteousness. I wanted to bring the sacrifice prescribed by the rabbis as penance for my obliviousness to the Sabbath. And, I thought, the best thing about me, really the only good thing about me, is that, when I was a child, I read for the sheer joy of losing myself in books, not so that I would know things or become the sort of person who had read this or that. I thought that I might be able to read the Torah that way.

Reading the way a child reads, it has since dawned on me, has always been part of the conversion experience. Saint Augustine, as he lay weeping on the ground, struggling to be saved, unwilling to be saved, wretched at the thought of his wretchedness, "the frivolity of frivolous aims, the futility of futile pursuits," imagined that he heard a child's voice nearby—"perhaps a boy or a girl, I do not know." The voice sang a ditty, over and over: "Pick it up and read, pick it up and read." So he did. He picked it up and read the first passage his eyes lit upon in the book that he had brought with him out to the garden, which contained the epistles of Paul: *Not in dissipation and drunkenness, nor in debauchery and lewdness, nor in arguing and jealousy; but put on the Lord Jesus Christ, and make no provision for the flesh or the gratification of your desires.* And he read no further, for "the light of certainty" flooded his heart, and "all dark shades of doubt fled away."

Where does the text get its power to redeem? Augustine doesn't say; rather, he deftly sets us up for this passage, so that we see its immediate relevance for the dissipated, lustful man he represents himself as being. The Kabbalists had an answer, though. The Torah, they thought, is not just a message left by the divine author. It is not the mere traces of Revelation. Nor are its words the mere instruments of God's will. The Torah is the actual emanation of God, Revelation itself, the will of God incarnate. To put it philosophically, the Torah has an ontological reality. It has Being—the ultimate being.

And Being, as any philosophy major knows, has Presence. And so reading becomes a way of being in the presence of—of being intimate with—God. From this point of view, it doesn't matter what the words say, which is why the Kabbalists felt free to break words down into letters, then transpose the letters into wildly nonbiblical and non-Talmudic myths, involving a God who withdraws into himself and primordial universes that shatter and heavenly spheres that function as God's avatars. *Reading* is how you overcome your loneliness and grow close to God. *Interpreting* and *acting on your words* come later. The Sabbath is what gives you time to read the Book, and what you read in the Book is that you must keep the Sabbath. Each provides the necessary technology for the movement of return.

PART SIX

Scenes of Instruction

1.

I HAD ALWAYS BEEN A GOOD STUDENT, BUT A STUPID ONE AT THE SAME time. I mastered material, but never actually learned anything. I was too busy displaying academic excellence. The history I would remember, the novels that would remain real to me, the languages I learned to the point where I could wrap my tongue around their strange diphthongs, I grappled with by myself, alone in a room. Only then could I read with a concentration that resembled pleasure, freed from the anxiety aroused by a group and a person with authority to grade me.

The first time I was invited to study with the Park Slope congregation on a Saturday afternoon, I felt a paper-sharp slice of shame. Me, a serious student of literary theory, reduced to a synagogue adult-education class! But I knew that I would go, and I did. The study session did not reassure me. Armed with a photocopy of a short piece of Talmud, we plunged right in.

No text is less reader-friendly than the Talmud. Even the pages look like fortresses, with blocks of text nestled inside blocks of commentary ringed by more blocks of commentary. At the center of certain pages lies the first word of the passage under discussion, set apart by an ornate fence. The Talmud is Law, but to read it as law is a mistake. Although it furnishes later rabbis with the raw material of legal rulings, it is not a law book. It offers no general principles, is not thematically organized, and makes no effort to sum things up. You analyze all the exceptions to a rule, for instance, before you find anything that articulates that rule, or you are forced to deduce the main principle from its exceptions.

Nor is the Talmud theology. Judaism lacks doctrinal discourse in the Christian mode, and Jews didn't start writing expository prose until rather late in their history, when they began trying to fit into Christian society. Rather, Judaism embeds its values deep within unexpected places: in rituals, in legends, in arcane legal and ethical discussions. When you first encounter what passes for law and theology in the Talmud, it's likely to strike you as scattershot and shockingly concrete (the anti-Semitic terms are nitpicky and hairsplitting). The rabbis fretted about matters of the utmost apparent triviality. The Sabbath tractate is consumed by the proper time for getting a haircut on Friday afternoon, the carrying of quantities of liquid that you could hold in your cheek on the Sabbath, how to deal with emissions of gonorrheal pus on the Sabbath. One result of this weird mode of transmission is that it's left up to the Jew to derive the principles of a Jewish life for him- or herself. (The Jewish philosopher Max Kadushin says that Judaism doesn't have ideas per se; it has "value-concepts," which are by definition non-definable, because they are embodied in actions or statements about actions.)

What the Talmud does is ask questions. It's an exercise in the confection of bizarre hypotheticals that probe the scope and limitations of every legal or ethical proposition. Why this and not that? If this is true, how do we know that it's true? Is it true in this case, in that one, in both, in neither? If you approach the Talmud expecting something like, say, the United States civil code, you will be lost. The Talmud is more like the minutes of legal-study sessions, except that the hundreds of scholars involved in these sessions were enrolled in a seminar that went on for more than a millennium, raising every conceivable aspect of life and ritual, in a free-form, associative order.

There's something wonderfully literary about all this. You rarely find in the Talmud a statement that has not been placed (with historical accuracy or not) in some ancient rabbi's mouth. And every so often you find parables—midrashim—like little jewels in the text. None is longer than a line or two and all are delivered with brusque non-explanatoriness, as if the rabbis had channeled Franz Kafka or Jorge Luis Borges (which they did if you believe, as Borges did, that every moment in history is pregnant with all those that follow it). Insofar as midrashim may be adduced to illustrate some legal principle, more often than not they contradict whatever law seems to be laid down. Professors in graduate history programs preach against the dangers of presentism, the habit of seeing the past through the lens of the present. There is no need to worry about that with the Talmud. It is the ultimate Brechtian instrument of alienation. You couldn't assimilate it to anything you knew if you wanted to. This is one way in which reading the Talmud is a spiritual discipline. It tests your ability to survive complete disorientation.

The first passage that we studied happened to be the first passage of the Talmud itself. "From when should we fulfill the obligation to recite the *Shema* in the evenings?" asks the Mishnah, the oldest layer of the text, which was compiled in the early third century. "From the time that the priests came in to eat their portion." Why start with the Shema? Why ask about the time? When did the priests eat their portion? Why were we talking about priests, anyway, when the rabbis did not codify law until after Temple worship had become a thing of the past? We asked these questions. Our rabbi told us to wait.

There would be no answers—not to the questions being asked, anyway. The Gemara, the next layer of commentary, seemed to acknowledge our confusion when it asked, "To what is this rabbi referring . . . and why does he teach the law regarding the evening first?" But all hope of clarification vanished with the next line: "Let him teach the law of the morning first!" This would not do. I wanted pre-

ambles, introductory lectures, supplementary readings. All we were
doing was translating and being baffled by what we found. On the
other hand, I didn't want to stop. As we homed in on the absurdly
concrete points of dispute, we were drawn into a peculiar intimacy. It
was as if we had entered a seminar room that had been cryogenically
frozen millennia ago, its questions and answers still hanging in the air.
Nothing could be mistaken for conclusive. Everything that had been
argued could be defrosted and argued again. The room we studied in
had a dusty, living-room feel; light sank in from the windows, and
swept slowly across the dark wooden floor. We felt no pressure to
hurry and finish as the Sabbath afternoons crawled on.

It was an innovation of the ancient rabbis to place the obligation
to study above any other commandment. An early Mishnah outlines
mitzvoth rewarded both in this world and in the next—charity, care
of one's parents—then declares that studying, *talmud Torah,* equals
them all. The religious Jew is to study Torah for the sake of studying
Torah, *Torah lishmah*. The ingenuity of the edict, I realized, was that it
relieved you of the obligation to be qualified. You studied because you
had to study, and those who taught had to take you as a student, and
it didn't matter whether you were an idiot or a savant. This is not to
say that brilliance doesn't matter in the Jewish world—nobody
swoons over genius as deliriously as a Jew—but, at the same time,
being unbrilliant was no excuse. Everyone had to study, and any day
was a good day to start.

Indeed, the rabbis loved to tell tales of scholarly giants who never
opened a book until well into middle age. One day, I found myself sitting cross-legged on the floor at another Saturday-afternoon study
session. It was a *seudah shlishit,* the "third meal" of the Sabbath, a light
dinner meant to compensate for the feast of Saturday lunch. We sat in
a circle in the rabbi's garden apartment in the North Slope. I sipped a
glass of scotch. The rabbi, a strangely Victorian figure with a long red
beard, came from Scotland, and loved to press single malts on his congregants. He was a young, shy man with a soft, singsongy voice. When
he taught, his voice went up at the end of sentences, as if he wondered
whether you had followed his meaning.

By then I had a crush on him and was jealous of any attention he paid to anyone else. I hogged the conversation, which was about a midrash. Its subject was Rabbi Akiva, who, the story goes, worked as a shepherd and liked to express an elaborate disdain for scholars. Then—at the age of forty—he was taken up by the daughter of a wealthy man who married him against the wishes of her father, but only on the condition that he go to a yeshiva and study. The father cut her off; she had to sell her hair to pay Akiva's way through school. Twenty-four years later, Akiva had become the greatest rabbi of his generation.

I was starting to know better by now, but old habits persisted. I had quibbles to offer, exegetical subtleties to point out. The argumentative techniques of the ancient rabbis remained as obscure to me as hieroglyphics, but I felt as though deep in my body I already knew what they had to say. I wanted to communicate this sensation of déjà vu, but I didn't know how. Instead, I raised my hand a lot. After a while, the rabbi began to ignore me with a gentle, congenial indifference. After a while longer, he refused to turn his head in my direction.

Some time after it finally occurred to me to put my hand back down, I closed my eyes and drifted into a daydream. I saw the group of us deep in a forest, floating in a boat on the surface of a lake that was small but deep. The rabbi cast down a bucket and brought up water full of weird plants and fish. He reached in and drew out, one by one, a plant, a fish, a stone. He showed them to us and told us about them. Their forms were not the least bit recognizable, and suddenly we understood that we had reentered an earlier period of evolution, a lost order of time. We were his followers; he was our leader—he might have been Jesus, or Akiva, or any other charismatic master. The Talmud was not a text, I thought. It was an umbilical cord. It linked us to a primordial scene of instruction.

This was surely no more than the self-protective tuning-out of a person who knows she has embarrassed herself, but I was also realizing something. The Talmud was not a text in the formal sense in which I had previously understood the word. The Talmud was an organism, circulating blood between the present and the deepest past. It was the word received at Sinai—the Oral Torah, it is called, to distinguish it from Scripture, the Written Torah—carried forward in the flesh. "Moses received [Oral] Torah from Sinai and transmitted it to Joshua, and Joshua to the elders, and the elders to the prophets, and the prophets transmitted it to the men of the Great Assembly" is the opening verse of *Pirkei Avot,* the "Ethics of the Fathers." Body carried the Oral Torah to body. It was no accident that the norms of Torah study involve physical proximity. Students study in pairs, in a *hevruta;* discipleship—*shimmush*—to a sage amounts not to apprenticeship but to a total recasting of the disciple in the mold of the mentor.

How did this work? By means of an almost unthinkable intimacy. How intimate was this intimacy? Go and learn, as the Talmud says. "Rabbi Akiva said: 'Once I went into an outhouse with Rabbi Joshua, and I learned from him three things. I learned that you don't sit east and west but north and south; I learned that you defecate not standing but sitting; and I learned that it is proper to wipe with the left hand and not with the right.' Ben Azzai said to him, 'How did you dare take such liberties with your master?' He replied, 'It was a matter of Torah, and I was required to learn.' "

Even defecating in the company of your teacher didn't go far enough. The Talmud describes this scene of ultimate education: "Rabbi Kahana once went and hid under Rab's bed. He heard him chatting [with his wife] and joking and doing everything he was supposed to do. Kahana said to Rab: 'You'd think your mouth never sipped this dish before!' Rab said to him: 'Kahana, what are you doing here? Get out! This is rude!' Kahana replied: 'It is a matter of Torah, and I want to learn.' "

Every level of the Talmud affirms the necessity of staying securely attached to your teachers—and I mean "attached" as in attachment theory, "attached" as infants are to their mothers. When I reread that first passage of Talmud, I concluded that the rabbis of the Gemara cared much less about parsing the Law than about making sure that the chain of oral transmission had not been broken. They asked not what but who. Who stated a certain dictum first? Who might have contradicted him? How do we decide who's right? Do their opinions have biblical warrant; that is, can they be defended by verses in Scripture, which, of course, would take them back to Moses? Those sages whose opinions are being quoted—how long ago did they live? Which generation of sages did they belong to? The first? Then their views have great weight. The fifth or sixth? Proportionally less weight. The fewer years that have lapsed between a rabbinic master and Moses, the more likely it is that he can be counted on to have known what he was talking about.

The Talmud, in other words, is like a giant game of Telephone. That umbilical cord does double duty as a telephone cord. When we study the Talmud, even when we don't understand what we're reading, we listen in on the crackles and the static and the distant heartbeats of something garbled and important that goes by the name of Revelation.

2.

AMONG ALL THE OTHER THINGS that it is, the Sabbath is a scene of instruction. In Josephus's histories and in the Gospels, we already find tales of scribes reading the Torah aloud to Jews in synagogues on Saturdays. But that's just the most obvious way in which the Sabbath educates. The Sabbath is not just a purveyor of books (or the Book), though it's that, too. It's an all-encompassing educational technology, involving the body, the mind, and the soul. A religion, like any cultural artifact that is not genetically predetermined, needs a way to pass its beliefs and practices from one generation to the next. The Sabbath—daylong, regular, putting entire families in physical contact with figures of authority who can both speak about and personally embody the religious way of life—is that kind of mechanism. In fact, it may be the most effective machine for the reproduction of values anyone has ever come up with.

For it is a process of total immersion. The Sabbath addresses itself to the whole student, imparting not just knowledge or information but also moral edification, behavioral example, ritual training, and

religio-political consciousness. By keeping the Sabbath, or so it supposedly went in the olden days, we learned what to do and what not
to do, how to carry ourselves, and how to relate to parents or authority figures, and from all these intangible lessons we could deduce no-
tions of holiness or at least the good. The Puritan Sabbath, for
instance, properly attended to, studious and decorous, was an exercise
in self-control, and it was meant to effect a "reformation of manners"
throughout seventeenth- and eighteenth-century England and America. Rid the lands of sports, plays, alehouses, drunken revelries, and
maypole dancing on the Sabbath, they thought; replace them with
soberness, churchgoing, sermons, Bible study, self-scrutiny, time discipline, and acts of charity; and you'd soon find yourself in the holiest
(and, as Max Weber would point out in *The Protestant Ethic and the
Spirit of Capitalism,* the wealthiest) of nations, surrounded by the most
dignified and reverential of fellow citizens.

This is not to give short shrift to the unquantifiable hours of
straight textbook learning that have gone on—and still go on—on
the Sabbath. If you are at all like me, you grew up thinking of Sunday
schools (or Saturday schools, for that matter) as infinitely tedious
places, taught by prigs eager to produce more prigs. (I spent as much
as possible of my teenage religious education behind the synagogue
with fellow would-be rebels while leaning on a cinder-block wall,
one foot up in that "fuck you" way.) You think that, in part, because
of the satirical or dark depictions of the Sabbath and its pedagogy
written by nineteenth-century novelists still read today, such as
Charles Dickens, Mark Twain, and Laura Ingalls Wilder (who wrote
in the twentieth century about her childhood in the nineteenth). In
Little House in the Big Woods (1932), Wilder describes her grandfather's
and great-aunts' and great-uncles' Sunday schooling in the 1820s:
They kept their eyes fixed on the preacher, afraid to turn their heads
to look out the window; ate a cold lunch; and after lunch studied their
catechism till the sun went down. Charles Dickens's *Little Dorrit*
(1855–1857), probably the most anti-Sabbatarian novel in history,
opens in London on a gloomy Sunday evening, when "maddening

church bells" were clanging and there was "nothing for the spent toiler to do, but to compare the monotony of his seventh day with the monotony of his six days, think what a weary life he led, and make the best of it—or the worst, according to the probabilities." The dour cityscape leads the novel's hero, Arthur Clenham, to reflect on the Sundays of his youth, and his Sunday education, conducted at first by his obsessively Puritanical mother: She "would sit all day behind a Bible—bound, like her own construction of it, in the hardest, barest, and straitest boards." (Naturally, she turns out not to have been his mother at all, but a wicked impostor.) Later he was subjected to a "picket of teachers" who marched him to chapel "three times a day, morally handcuffed to another boy" so he could listen to "indigestible sermons" that he would have happily traded "for another ounce or two of inferior mutton at his scanty dinner in the flesh."

Mark Twain, in his 1875 "Story of the Good Little Boy," offered up the opposite spectacle—that of Jacob Blivens, a model boy who "never was late at Sabbath school," "wouldn't play marbles on Sunday," had "read all the Sunday-school books," and "had a noble ambition to be put in a Sunday-school book." Naturally, nothing in Jacob's life turns out the way it does in Sunday-school books: Jacob rushes to the rescue of a blind man who, instead of blessing him, cracks him over the head with a cane. The boy tries to warn some boys in a sailboat that they're breaking the Sabbath and will drown; instead, he nearly drowns himself. The story ends when he is blown to bits by a nitroglycerine can meant to be tied to the tail of a dog while he is admonishing the boys who are about to tie it.

These works reflect the rise, in the nineteenth century, and on both sides of the Atlantic, of a sardonic anti-Sabbatarianism. It emerged partly as a response to the unusual strictness of the English and American Sunday compared to Sundays elsewhere in the world; partly out of the irritated sense that Sabbath legislation had become hypocritical, anti–working class, and antimodern; and partly because of a growing revulsion at moral and religious legislation of any kind. English and American Sabbath sentiment and lawmaking had waxed and waned in the two centuries since the heyday of Puritan power in the seventeenth century, but its social effects and legislative apparatus remained largely in place. In England, for instance, decades after Oliver Cromwell and his largely Puritan Parliament had been ousted from power and the English monarchy and the anti-Sabbatarian Anglican Church had been restored, the average citizen felt that to engage in, or permit, sports and recreation on Sunday went against the will of God. Sunday travel and retail trade were also prohibited. Many in the middle classes kept the day in the Puritan manner, with minimal heat and hot food and few activities other than praying and reading holy texts. Samuel Johnson, for instance—who as an adult became an ardent defender of a less severe Sabbath—recollected the Sundays of his childhood as a grim time when "my mother confined me" and "made me read *The Whole Duty of Man*," a dull devotional work outlining man's responsibility to man and God, "from a great part of which I could derive no instruction."

By the mid-eighteenth century, British Sunday legislation had relaxed its grip, especially in the cities, where it regulated only the hours of service and left the rest of the day to the population's discretion; even in the countryside, where magistrates still forced people into churches and forbade trade on Sunday, the middle classes began to brighten up the day with a large midday meal. (The Sunday activities of the urban upper and lower classes in that period are vividly described in a pamphlet published in 1755 by one Thomas Legg, titled "Low Life, or One Half of the World Knows Not How the Other Half Lives." Sunday, to Legg's rakish eye, gave the upper classes extra time to engage in their usual activities, that is, drink, make merry, and get fleeced; gave the criminal classes an extra opportunity to fleece; and gave the serving classes a reason to work harder than usual. Among those who broke the Sabbath in the early hours of Sunday morning were the rich, who frequented "Gaming-Tables, Night-Houses, Bawdy Houses, Geneva Shops, and other Places of Resort which are contrary to Acts of Parliament." Among those who violated the Fourth Commandment during the day were "Taylors, Shoe-Makers, Stay-Makers, Mantua Makers, Milliners, Glove-Washers,

Hoop-Petticoat and Capuchin Makers," as well as prostitutes, barbers, and, of course, servants and other service providers: "Footmen in the Back-Back Kitchens of Nobility and Gentry, cleaning of such Plate as will be necessary for the ornamenting the Buffet and Side-Board"; "Poor Women and Lame Men, whose Bread depends chiefly on sweeping the Passages to Churches, Chapels, and Meetings"; "Shoe-Blackers and Hackney Coachmen"; "Gardeners who live at Gentle-man's Houses near London, mowing and sweeping the Grass-Plats, and rolling the Gravel-Walks, to make them fit for the Reception of their Masters and Mistresses.")

Sabbath legislation resurged in England and America at the beginning of the nineteenth century, largely because of the rise of evangelicism on both continents—Nonconformism in England (the Nonconformists did not conform to the principles of the official Church of England) and the Second Great Awakening in the United States (from which we got revivalism and camp meetings). Sabbatari-ans formed societies (today we'd call them lobbies). Parliamentarians and senators commissioned studies and introduced bills to promote, as one such bill put it, "the Better Observance of the Lord's Day."

In dispute were the new technologies and cultural institutions that were transforming the rhythms of daily life—trains, post offices, and museums—and the degree to which they would be subject to Sunday regulation. Factions representing business interests battled factions representing religious interests over such matters as Sunday railroad travel, Sunday postal service, Sunday trade, Sunday newspapers, and Sunday amusements.

In 1810, the U.S. Congress passed legislation requiring mail to be delivered and post offices opened on Sundays, spurring a furious backlash among ministers and congregations and initiating one of the biggest political battles in U.S. history. The historian Richard R. John writes, "The protest was unprecedented. Never before had the federal government interfered so directly with the rhythms of everyday life. Never before had so many Americans formally challenged the authority of their elected representatives to legislate on matters touching on deeply held religious beliefs." In 1852, a Kulturkampf broke out in London over the Crystal Palace, an enormous glass and iron building in Hyde Park that housed fourteen thousand exhibitors during a Great Exhibition celebrating technology and progress. The Sabbatarians ultimately won the fight to keep it closed on Sunday, which so infuriated the anti-Sabbatarians that they agitated for opening the British Museum on Sundays and allowing military bands to play in the parks on Sunday afternoons. A similar battle was fought over the Metropolitan Museum in New York City.

Progressives and radicals in both countries (including Karl Marx, during his early years as a journalist reporting on English affairs) began demanding that the worshipful Sunday be replaced by the educationally and culturally enriching kind, arguing that this would especially benefit immigrants (in the United States) and the working classes (in both countries). Activists founded societies to promote the openings of museums and libraries on Sunday and to encourage Sunday lecture series and Sunday concerts. Sabbatarians accused those anti-Sabbatarians of trying to foster a "Continental Sabbath," the laxer Sabbath of Catholic Europe, where Sunday afternoon, at least, was a time for recreation. In the United States, if you were an Anglo-Saxon Protestant who happened to dwell in a city where immigrants also lived, you might see them keeping that kind of Sabbath—strolling about, laughing, drinking, enjoying street theater—and it smacked suspiciously of foreignness. The Sabbatarians bolstered their counter-argument by claiming that stronger Sunday laws would help the working classes by protecting them from Sunday labor. The anti-Sabbatarians replied that Sabbath laws were no substitute for real labor legislation, especially the kind that limited the length of the working day and week. They attacked the Sabbatarians as hypocrites for outlawing Sunday fun while allowing Sunday drinking, for exempting their servants from the Fourth Commandment, and for justifying several other forms of service as acts of necessity and mercy. Each side worked up its own clichés. Sabbatarians painted nostalgic portraits of idyllic Sundays in quaint villages. Anti-Sabbatarians made ample use of the figure of the bored child fidgeting the day away, in the thrall of some pedantic Sunday schoolmaster.

Many such children surely existed; they may well have been in the majority. But it's worth remembering that it was the Sunday pedagogical tradition that made it possible to envision more revolutionary kinds of Sunday education. When Sunday schools first came into existence in England, to take an example, they helped to transform the lower classes they served. Set up largely by the intellectuals and activists of the evangelical revival of the late eighteenth century (many of whom later became abolitionists) in order to keep the children of the desperately poor from breaking the Sabbath by running wild on the streets, these schools gave many such children the only education they'd ever have. Sometimes they gave it to their parents and grown siblings, too.

The Sunday schools for the poor came along at a time when such opportunities were rare, at least for children whose parents couldn't spare their help or wages long enough to send them to weekday schools, or couldn't afford to send them for more than a year or two. The historian Thomas Laqueur, in a study called *Religion and Respectability: Sunday Schools and Working Class Culture, 1780–1850*, argues that these schools offered not just escape from poverty but also a venue for what we would now call community organizing, as well as job training for graduates who often began illustrious careers by teaching in the schools. Some of them would go on to become the leaders and educators of emerging working-class political parties. The early Sunday school was a nursery of piety, yes, but it could also be a cradle of working-class self-awareness.

Not all of them proselytized, either. Many of the early schools were interdenominational—a lack of funds required them to affiliate with all the churches in town, not just with one—which meant that they had to refrain from advancing a particular doctrine. Too strict a theology could kindle controversy. Their mission, instead, was literacy. Most schools taught at least two of the three Rs, reading and writing, and some taught the third, arithmetic; the texts studied were catechisms and Scripture, but the skills taught could be transferred to other endeavors. (Schools that didn't teach the basics soon found themselves short of students.) Going to school one day a week wasn't as good as going five or six days a week, as the other working-class schools (the "charity schools") required. Nonetheless, as Laqueur points out, the Sunday school featured a very long day—three to five hours—and students went for an average of four years, and the Sunday-school movement wound up having "a significant impact on the creation of mass literacy in nineteenth-century England."

Skeptics dismiss nineteenth-century British Sunday-school instruction as opium for the masses, or, more precisely, as a cynical means of divorcing peasants and artisans from their casual, seasonal approach to labor by teaching them a work ethic underscored by a fear of damnation. The schools' ambition, by these lights, was to turn rural folk into industrial drones through what one nineteenth-century historian called "religious terrorism." The cautionary tales of bad boys and girls who met dire fates that were found in the Sunday-school primers amounted to "psychological atrocities," the socialist historian E. P. Thompson wrote in his 1963 *Making of the English Working Class.* Thompson quoted the author of a "Satanic" book called *Philosophy of Manufactures* (1835) that offered this advice to factory owners: Make sure that workers receive a sound spiritual education, because "the neglect of moral discipline" leads to "the disorder of the general system, the irregularities of the individual machines, the waste of time and material."

The founders of the Sunday schools, however, saw themselves as reformers fighting for a progressive cause. Everyone from bishops to local squires opposed them, and they had to refute the widespread belief that educating the poor would turn them into dissatisfied rabble-rousers, otherwise known, in a reference to the French Revolution, as Jacobins. The reformer Hannah More, for instance, told worried farmers in the town of Cheddar that Sunday school would improve, not harm, their laborers' behavior: "I . . . said that I had a little plan which I hoped would secure their orchards from being robbed, and their rabbits from being shot, their game from being stolen, and *might* lower the Poor Rates." But privately she told a friend (William Wilberforce, the politician who led the British abolitionist movement) that she came up with these arguments only to secure the support of a rich local "Despot" and all the other "petty Tyrants" of Cheddar who feared that bringing religion to the poor would make them "lazy and useless."

Once gathered in the schools, students and teachers organized ambitious programs to improve their quality of life. They formed sick societies (a rough form of health insurance), benefit societies (unemployment insurance), and funeral societies (life insurance, of sorts), along with "clothing clubs" (to which people donated their used clothing) and employment exchanges (that is, communal employment agencies). Because the schools were voluntary rather than compulsory, they were obliged to be enjoyable, and alotted more time to festivities—outings and graduation ceremonies and holiday parties— than ordinary schools did, even if the fun was unduly prim for its day (Sunday-school celebrations tended to feature milk instead of beer, a more popular refreshment). The act of dressing up for Sunday school could open a student's eyes to a more salutary way of life. Laqueur quotes Charles Shaw, a pottery worker whose attendance at Sunday school led to him to become a preacher:

> I got a washing that morning such as I had not time to get on other mornings. I had poor enough clothing to put on, but my eldest sister always helped me in my toilet on Sunday mornings, and my hair got brushed and combed and oiled [with scented oil]. . . . Amidst these unfriendly and perilous circumstances, the influences of the Sunday school stood me in good stead. It was not so much that I understood the evil about me and saw into its baleful depths, as that I had an inward influence which gave me an opposite bias and always made me think of the Sunday school.

There were surely many stultifying Sunday-school teachers to go along with all the bored students. But the teachers of the Sunday schools for the poor seem to have been capable of providing a different kind of experience and of communicating less conventional and non-condescending ideas to their students. Charles Shaw says that Sunday school taught him about "two different worlds—one belonging to God and Father I read about in Sunday school every Sunday; and the other belonging to the rich men, to manufacturers, to squires and nobles, and all kinds of men of authority. These I supposed made the world of men what it was, through sheer badness in treatment of all who had work." George Holyoake, a socialist who invented the term *secularist,* learned logic and mathematics and cooperative socialism from his teachers at a Unitarian Sunday school. Rowland Detrosier, a working-class radical, started out as the superintendent of a Swedenborgian Sunday school in Hulme, England. He taught himself natural history, astronomy, electricity, and mechanics, among other subjects, because his students wanted to learn about them. "Let our Sunday schools become the UNIVERSITIES OF THE POOR," he declared.

These Sunday schools didn't stay interdenominational for long; bitter jockeying among the different churches prevented that. They didn't stay under the control of lay teachers, either. By the middle of the nineteenth century, few of the schools still taught writing; religious officials with a stricter construction of Sabbath propriety thought that was breaking the Sabbath. Nonetheless, the idea of a Sunday school as a source of values different from the ones observed the rest of the week lingered on. As long as religious Sunday schools had a working-class flavor, secular and political Sunday schools—labor-union schools, communist schools—failed to thrive. When Sunday schools got too righteous, socialists in both England and America seized the opportunity to found a slew of what one happy student called rebel factories, complete with songs, arts and crafts, games, and plays that taught lessons on capitalism, exploitation, and worker solidarity. Few of these schools survived the Red scares of the 1920s, but in their heyday there were dozens in England and nearly a hundred in the United States.

3.

AS THE SABBATH STARTED to shed its religious meanings, it began to be seen as a day of personal and social improvement. This, too, was in part an effect of the association between the Sabbath and pedagogy. If you wanted to identify the remains of a Sabbatarian sensibility in our view of the weekend today, you might start with the sense that we are obliged to use it to better our condition. We think of Saturday and Sunday as time not merely for resting but for trying to become the kind of people that work prevents us from being. We catch up on our reading. We try to get our children to spend some time playing out of doors. All this was learned in the nineteenth century, when people began to reconceive of Sunday variously as an opportunity to refresh their parched spirits, to return to a natural world from which they felt increasingly cut off, and to rediscover lost connections with those around them.

In his writings on the Sabbath, Dickens didn't only attack Sabbatarian hypocrisies; he also advocated the use of Sunday for restorative outings, and in so doing helped release a torrent of literature arguing that Sunday should be a day for promoting mental well-being and improving moral character. Call this the Hygienic Sabbath. In 1836, during his time as a reporter on parliamentary affairs, Dickens published a pamphlet attacking a piece of proposed legislation that would have strengthened Sunday closing laws. In the pamphlet, he contrasts the stifling Sundays of the urban poor, who get bored and drunk and commit crimes because they are kept from exercise and recreation by Sunday-closing laws, and the expansive Sundays of those who are free to enjoy the sun, the wind, and Sunday outings. Dickens's description of one healthful Sunday is by far the most vivid of its kind, so I'll quote it at length:

Here and there, so early as six o'clock, a young man and woman in their best attire, may be seen hurrying along on their way to the house of some acquaintance, who is included in their scheme of pleasure for the day; from whence, after stopping to take "a bit of breakfast," they sally forth, accompanied by several old people, and a whole crowd of young ones, bearing large hand-baskets full of provisions, and Belcher handkerchiefs done up in bundles, with the neck of a bottle sticking out at the top, and closely-packed apples

bulging out at the sides,—and away they hurry along the streets
leading to the steam-packet wharfs, which are already plentifully
sprinkled with parties bound for the same destination. Their good
humour and delight know no bounds—for it is a delightful morning, all blue over head, and nothing like a cloud in the whole sky;
and even the air of the river at London Bridge is something to them,
shut up as they have been, all the week, in close streets and heated
rooms. . . . Away they go, joking and laughing, and eating and drinking, and admiring everything they see, and pleased with everything
they hear, to climb Windmill Hill, and catch a glimpse of the rich
corn-fields and beautiful orchards of Kent; or to stroll among the
fine old trees of Greenwich Park, and survey the wonders of
Shooter's Hill and Lady James's Folly; or to glide past the beautiful
meadows of Twickenham and Richmond, and to gaze with a delight
which only people like them can know, on every lovely object in the
fair prospect around. Boat follows boat, and coach succeeds coach,
for the next three hours; but all are filled, and all with the same kind
of people—neat and clean, cheerful and contented.

If today we think of the weekend as a time for communing with
nature, that, too, was the doing of nineteenth-century writers. In the
hands of poets, novelists, and intellectuals, the Sabbath became a lyri-
cal and pastoral notion, a weekly haven from the burgeoning industrial order. You might think of the turn toward nature as a swerve
away from theology, and it was, but since the swerve was made under
the sway of poets, God was never far from their thoughts. Nature, to
them, was God's true abode, and they considered gamboling or wandering outdoors a holier pastime than confining their limbs to a pew
or desk. "Some keep the Sabbath going to Church—," wrote Emily
Dickinson in 1861. "I keep it, staying at Home— / With a Bobolink
for a Chorister— / And an Orchard, for a Dome—." And so: "instead
of getting to Heaven at last— / I'm going all along."

If you were going to trace the natural Sabbath back to one man
in particular (a dubious exercise, I know), it would probably be Jean-

Jacques Rousseau, the autobiographer, novelist, philosopher, and political theorist who simultaneously inspired the French Revolution,
the Romantic return-to-nature movement, and various forms of radical pedagogy. "Childhood is unknown" is how Rousseau opened his
prescient if rather strange book *Emile, or On Education* (strange because of Rousseau's many strange opinions, such as his conviction that
children should not be allowed to read made-up stories). Rousseau's
views on pedagogy were the exact opposite of the Sabbatarian practice of it. The Puritans had treated children as little adults. They had
dressed their babes in grown-up clothes and taught them grown-up
theology and made them conform to grown-up manners, especially
in church. But Rousseau insisted that children amount to a foreign
species hidden in plain sight, with their own logic and modes of cognition. Moreover, child and nature are one, which means that child
and nature and God are one, too, and all are good. The child, closer to
nature than the adult, is holier than adults, too, since human institutions, including most forms of schooling, are unnatural and corrupt-
ing. Therefore, the place for children to learn about God is not in
church on Sunday, but out of doors. They can deduce his existence
from the workings of nature and thereby cultivate the divine within
themselves.

I should say that Rousseau never wrote about the Sabbath. Nor
did he keep it. If he had, I feel certain that he would have spent it
strolling through the countryside, investigating botanical specimens.
In the fifth of his *Reveries of a Solitary Walker,* for instance, Rousseau
described as the happiest period of his life two months spent on a remote island in a Swiss lake called, evocatively, Lake of Bienne (*Bienne*
evoking, to the French ear, *bien,* which means "well"), to which he
had fled after his books *Emile* and *The Social Contract* had been condemned by the French Parliament and his house pelted with stones.
On his island refuge, cut off from the outside world with all its demands, he engaged in the "precious *far niente,*" the doing of nothing,
and lost himself for hours each day in the study of blades of grass, bits
of moss, lichen.

Rousseau, in that essay, helped define the modern idea of time off. He sketched out the notion of a time out of time that, though not religious per se, is prelapsarian—that is, as whole and non-alienated as the time before Adam and Eve were exiled from the garden. "What, then, was this happiness, and in what did this joy consist?" asked Rousseau. Part of it was the relief of not having to live up to expectations, part of it was the delight of investigating flowers and plants, and part of it was giving himself over to reverie. But part of it had to do with a novel yet very old sense of time, time experienced as he imagined babies experience it, as plenitude and sensation and living in the moment. Grown-up time, Rousseau declared, is absent from itself. We fall into it as we fell from Eden, yet we never occupy it. We dwell in the past and the future but never in the present. At no one moment of existence is there anything "solid enough for the heart to attach itself to." But now, as he sat at the Lake of Bienne, sometimes rocking in a boat, sometimes waiting on the shore of the lake when the water happened to be rough, he rediscovered a way of being in time "that, as long as it lasts, could be called happy."

This was the first inkling of what I'd call the Romantic Sabbath, an unpressured, serendipitous, nostalgic experience of time in which the soul finds "a seat solid enough to rest itself there completely and to gather together all its being without needing to recall the past or to straddle the future." This idea was developed by William Wordsworth in his epic, *The Prelude* (1799–1805), the tale of how nature formed him as a poet—its full title is *The Prelude, or Growth of a Poet's Mind: An Autobiographical Poem*. In the poem, Wordsworth touches only glancingly on the Sabbath, but he has a great deal to say about time and how it shaped his identity, and the Sabbath plays a more important role than its brief mention would seem to imply.

Wordsworth begins the poem by fleeing the city for a stroll in the Lake Country, during which he tries to begin writing his great poem in his head. Instead of plunging in, he finds himself lounging in the shade of a tree, "slackening my thoughts by choice." He tries to start the poem again: "my soul / once more made trial of her strength."

Once again he fails. Finally, he realizes that he must cease his striving and accept the need for silence. He must not "bend the Sabbath of that time / To a servile yoke." Giving in to the Sabbath and the non-productivist side of his nature, to what his fellow Romantic John Keats called his negative capability, Wordsworth strays about "Voluptuously, through fields and rural walks"; he asks "no record of the hours, resigned / To vacant musing, unreproved neglect / Of all things, and deliberate holiday."

This "holiday" from the work of composition, this starting, stopping, then wandering off, will leave its stamp on *The Prelude,* which curls, shaggy and undulating, "mazy as a river," in critic Geoffrey Hartman's phrase, back and forth between present and past and through the twists and turns of Wordsworth's slow maturation. The "Sabbath of that time" is the moment (or perhaps the anti-moment) that allows the poet to break through to another order of time—"spots of time," he calls them elsewhere. In these spots, "our minds / Are nourished and invisibly repaired." As in, say, the psychoanalytic session (an idea not unaffected by Wordsworth, or at least by Romanticism), memories reawaken and joys and traumas are lived and felt again and understood perhaps for the first time.

Wordsworth, of course, is the quintessential nature poet; we imagine him hiking up mountains and strolling along shores in the English Lake District. And yet nature, for Wordsworth, had its own temporality as well as its own geography. E. P. Thompson would have called Wordsworth's idea of natural time "preindustrial," and it's true that in *The Prelude* Wordsworth makes much of a shepherd who lived an entirely seasonal life and worked "for himself, with choice / Of time, and place, and object." But Wordsworth's natural time was not merely the antithesis of industrial time. It had its own rhythms. At one point, for instance, Wordsworth gives heartfelt thanks that he had one of those free, outdoor, unsupervised childhoods that seems to have been rare even in the eighteenth century. Nature saved him, he writes, "from an evil which these days have laid / Upon the children of the land"—the evil of being tightly scheduled and oppressively supervised, "hourly watched, and noosed, / Each in his several melancholy walk / Stringed like a poor man's heifer at its feed, / Led through the lanes in forlorn servitude."

What is natural time like, for Wordsworth? It was like his late mother, he says, who in her maternal patience never demanded developmental milestones from her son, never "from the season asked / More than its timely produce; rather loved / The hours for what they are." Unnatural time, on the other hand, demands too much and destroys the soul. If natural time was female, unnatural time was male. Men are "the keepers of our time," who chain the young people in their charge to a predetermined path, "to the very road / Which they have fashioned would confine us down / Like engines." Accepting the "Sabbath of that time," then, means stopping unnatural time so as to create a moment for natural time, which allows one to expand and flourish according to its organic laws.

A less individualistic vision of the natural Sabbath—we could call this one the Communitarian Sabbath—comes to us from the novels of George Eliot, the nom de plume of Mary Ann Evans, who received an evangelical education but lost her religion when she entered the world of letters. Eliot had a broader vision of nature than Wordsworth did; for her, it was social as well as environmental and temporal, comprising not only the wilderness that lies beyond the reach of civilization but also the kind of community that is held together by organic bonds, by the ties of family, affection, and village economy. Eliot grew up in the countryside and possessed an encyclopedic understanding of the religious life of the small English town, and in her first novel, *Adam Bede* (1859), Eliot devotes a chapter to the sympathetic depiction of a village Sabbath in an English hamlet called Hayslope.

Adam Bede takes place sixty years before it was written, at the turn of the nineteenth century, when livelihoods still came from small farms and artisanal cottage industries. The Sabbath described in the novel probably seemed more pastoral in retrospect than at the time it occurred. When Eliot looked backward, she found "the deep-rooted folk memory of a 'golden age' or 'Merrie England,'" as E. P. Thompson put it, which "derives not from the notion that material goods were more plentiful in 1780 than in 1840 but from nostalgia for the pattern of work and leisure which obtained before the outer and inner disciplines of industrialism settled upon the working man." In Hayslope, the Sabbath does not descend from the heavens above; it ascends from the natural world below, "the cocks and hens," which "seemed to know" that it was Sunday "and made only crooning subdued noises," and the bull-dog, which looked "less savage, as if he would have been satisfied with a smaller bite than usual." The very sunshine "seemed to call all things to rest and not to labour."

Next to respond to the call of the Sunday sun are the people of the village, who primp for church then amble toward it, converging in the churchyard as the animals did in the farmyard. When the church service begins, the resonant spirits in the congregation swell with an imaginative capaciousness not available to them on any other day of the week. Adam Bede proves particularly susceptible to "the other deep feelings for which the church service was a channel . . . as a certain consciousness of our entire past and our imagined future blends itself with all our moments of keen sensibility." This Sunday sensibility does not grace only the spiritually gifted. It serves as the fulcrum of Hayslope life, and of the novel. Almost all of the important plot developments in *Adam Bede* occur on Sundays, when people have the time and the inclination to acknowledge and interact with one another. The hushed air of holiness that prevails when the church service ends turns a fractious town into a blessed community, for after that comes "the quiet rising, the mothers tying on the bonnets of the little maidens who had slept through the sermon, the fathers collecting the prayer-books, until all streamed out through the old archway into the green churchyard, and began their neighbourly talk, their simple civilities, and their invitations to tea."

In a letter written one Sunday about the Sabbath state of mind, George Eliot equated the religious experience with the poetic experience. Without religion, she said, we suffer the fate of "poor mortals" who wake up one morning and find "all the poetry in which their world was bathed only the evening before utterly gone—the hard angular world of chairs and tables and looking-glasses staring at them in

all its naked prose." Sunday cleared a space in which the imagination
might roam free—the social imagination as much as the individual
imagination; and the imagination, for Eliot, as for Wordsworth, is what
gives minds the power to tease out of ordinary life intimations of
beauty and a moral order.

The writer who best captured the Romantic Sabbath, though, to
my mind, is D. H. Lawrence—not a nineteenth-century writer, I
grant you, but one whose memory encompassed enough of the previous century to be worth including here. He, too, regretted
the vanishing of what he called the "Sunday world." In a scene in
Lawrence's novel *The Rainbow* (1915) largely based on his own childhood, Ursula Brangwen, his heroine, sadly contemplates the disappearance of "the old duality of life"—"wherein there had been a
week-day world of people and trains and duties and reports, and besides that a Sunday world of absolute truth and living mystery, of
walking upon the waters and being blinded by the face of the Lord,
of following the pillar of cloud across the desert and watching the
bush that crackled yet did not burn away."

Ursula's memories of her childhood Sundays combine both
Wordsworth's lyrically pastoral time and Eliot's blessed Sunday community in the figure of the happy member of the happy family. In
fact, Lawrence's description of a typical Sunday in Ursula's family offers such a perfect vision of human happiness that I can do no more
than quote it at length:

> Even at its stormiest, Sunday was a blessed day. Ursula woke to it
> with a feeling of immense relief. She wondered why her heart was so
> light. Then she remembered it was Sunday. A gladness seemed to
> burst out around her, a feeling of great freedom. The whole world
> was for twenty-four hours revoked, put back. Only the Sunday
> world existed.
>
> She loved the very confusion of the household. It was lucky if
> the children slept till seven o'clock. Usually, soon after six, a chirp
> was heard, a voice, an excited chirrup began, announcing the cre-

ation of a new day, there was a thudding of quick little feet, and the children were up and about, scampering in their shirts, with pink legs and glistening, flossy hair all clean from the Saturday's night bathing, their souls excited by their bodies' cleanliness.

As the house began to teem with rushing, half-naked clean children, one of the parents rose, either the mother, easy and slatternly with her thick, dark hair loosely coiled and slipping over one ear, or the father, warm and comfortable, with ruffled black hair and shirt unbuttoned at the neck. . . .

On this day of decorum, the Brangwen family went to church by the high-road, making a detour outside all the garden-hedge, rather than climb the wall into the churchyard. There was no law of this, from the parents. The children themselves were the wardens of the Sabbath decency, very jealous and instant with each other.

It came to be, gradually, that after church on Sundays the house was really something of a sanctuary, with peace breathing like a strange bird alighted in the rooms. Indoors, only reading and tale-telling and quiet pursuits, such as drawing, were allowed. Out of doors, all playing was to be carried on unobtrusively. If there were noise, yelling or shouting, then some fierce spirit woke up in the father and the elder children, so that the younger were subdued, afraid of being excommunicated.

The children themselves preserved the Sabbath. If Ursula in her vanity sang:

> "Il était un' bergère
> Et ron-ron-ron petit patapon,"

Theresa was sure to cry:
"*That's* not a Sunday song, our Ursula."

"You don't know," replied Ursula, superior. Nevertheless, she wavered. And her song faded down before she came to the end.

Because, though she did not know it, her Sunday was very precious to her. She found herself in a strange, undefined place, where her spirit could wander in dreams, unassailed.

4.
——

THIS IS WHAT I WAS LOOKING FOR, this "strange, undefined place" in the bosom of a joyful family wherein my spirit could safely wander, but since I had not read Lawrence, I could not describe this place or spot in time and had no idea how to find it. One Shabbat, I found myself sitting in the sun at the edge of a grassy courtyard inside a low brick mid-century apartment complex, watching toddlers toddle and their parents toddle with them. A couple from my synagogue, both classical musicians, were explaining the impossibility, for them, of keeping the Sabbath, given their performance schedules. Behind me, in a ground-floor apartment, members of the synagogue were eating a potluck Shabbat lunch. There was something magical about this courtyard, I thought. We had had Sabbath picnics in the park before, but they had never felt so idyllic. The seclusion of the space, the golden shimmer of the sun against the brown brick, gave it the aura of sanctuary.

I was also conscious of being bored. The wife was describing in obsessive detail the logistical difficulties of her life—of juggling motherhood, career, and Judaism. Not having entered the ranks of parents, I didn't actually care. I began to wonder whether by joining the shul I had prematurely entered a sort of spiritual suburb. The synagogue's membership consisted primarily of youngish couples. There was a subgroup of lesbians, some of them in their twenties, and another subgroup of female refugees from Orthodox Judaism, several of whom came from Brooklyn neighborhoods to the east and south of us. The two groups overlapped but were not identical. I belonged to neither of them. I found myself longing for lower Manhattan, the sharp if uncertain fashions of insecure people, the spontaneous parties, the round-robins of relationships from which people my age extract a "crowd." Suddenly, my return to Judaism struck me as an apprenticeship in being middle-aged.

I am always astonished, in retrospect, at how quickly the world collaborates with you once you have determined to run away from yourself. A few weeks after that moment, I met a man fifteen years older than me. He lived on the Upper West Side. He was an atheist, a comedy writer, a divorcé, a cynic. He had been middle-aged—by which he meant married—and didn't want to be again. His ex-wife was a writer, too, a well-known feminist, and together they had read, and talked about, and worked through the object lessons provided by writers I had encountered only as subject matter for term papers— Samuel Johnson, Mary Wollstonecraft, Antonio Gramsci. My new boyfriend was a man of the world. His jokes were allusive. He knew many people in the television industry personally. Being with someone so much older made me feel young again. He was funny and mean. He made me unhappy, and he made me laugh. He was elaborately patient with my newfound Judaism, by which I understood that he found it ridiculous, so that pretty soon I did, too. I stopped going to synagogue and moved to the Upper West Side.

5.

IT WAS FOUR YEARS before I began going to synagogue again on Saturdays, and when I did it was because I married (someone else) and moved to the suburbs, but, also, and more important, because I found another teacher. He was utterly different from my first teacher. Rabbi Paul (I'll call him) was a brilliant and widely disliked man. He had bold features and close-cropped curly black hair. He was Byronic in appearance and fearsome in his love of Jewish law, even though he had been a professor of philosophy before he became a pulpit rabbi, and did so largely because he had failed to get tenure.

Now that I spend so much time reading theology, people often ask me if I want to be a rabbi. I shudder at the thought. I can't imagine a more terrifying job. My answer is, go and read a very early novella by George Eliot called *The Sad Fortunes of the Reverend Amos Barton* (1857). The Reverend Amos Barton is a very good man but a very bad minister. His oratory resembles the bleatings of "a Belgian railway-horn." His predecessor in the parish generated "a certain amount of religious excitement," but now that feeling has died down. It is when he must preach to a gathering of poor folk that his deep pedestrianness shines through. Trained at Oxford, tenaciously pedantic, he simply can't think from the pauper's point of view. He can only deliver a dry sermon irrelevant to their lives. He knows full well that his congregants hold him in low esteem and probably contempt.

Rabbi Paul's unpopularity derived mainly from his uncompromising rigor in matters of ritual, but it also had a lot to do with his pastoral manner, or, rather, his unpastoral manner. He did not give sermons on Saturday mornings. He led graduate seminars. He would elicit opinions from members of his congregation about whatever portion of the Torah they were reading that week, and then, like the Socratic master he was trained to be, he'd derive from our innocent observations the deepest principles of religious thought. His speciality was the phenomenology of religion—the philosophical study of religion as experience, rather than as a set of claims that can be proved to be true or false. He adored Maurice Merleau-Ponty, but he told us to read Rabbi Abraham Joshua Heschel, who was less difficult and more Jewish. (The book he had us begin with was *The Sabbath*.)

Rabbi Paul's rhetorical style bored some and piqued others. I loved it. But this wasn't what got his congregants most riled up. Their complaint had to do with the way he reacted when someone gave an answer that he didn't like. Puritan preachers may have thundered, but clergymen today do not. Theological mandates no longer dictate the laws of the land. Religion, in our liberal pluralistic society, competes humbly with other lifestyle choices. Today, it is incumbent upon a minister to boost the members of his or her church, not to humiliate them. He or she stresses a God of self-actualization, not a God who shames and judges.

Rabbi Paul, however, shamed and judged. Not so much our moral failings as our intellectual ones. We gave dumb answers to his questions. We couldn't see where he was trying to go. We lacked original religious minds. To some congregant's halting guess about what gem the rabbi wished him to unearth in a dusty verse, he'd reply, "No! Next?" Had we not read the Torah portion? Had we not seen that the dying Abraham makes the eldest servant of his house put his hand under Abraham's thigh and swear to him that he will not let Isaac,

Abraham's son, choose a wife from among the Canaanites? Had we not asked ourselves what "under his thigh" meant, exactly? It meant the genitals, of course. *Put your hand on my penis:* Didn't that strike us as an odd form for a vow to take?

Well, yes, it did. But it was the standard form for vows in the ancient world. But what did it mean? *What did it mean?* Had we never asked ourselves why there are so many rules about sexuality in the Torah? Were our forefathers nothing more than unenlightened prudes? Had they simply never considered the advantages of sexual liberation? It seemed to Rabbi Paul that they had, and had rejected it. Consider the content of the vow the servant is asked to make: He is to swear that he will choose the right wife for Abraham's son. She is not to be Canaanite, which is to say, licentious. She is to be from Abraham's family, which is to say, decent. It seemed to Rabbi Paul that our forefathers did not fail to appreciate the terrible, necessary power of sexuality. Consider the almost baroque suspense that dominates several chapters in Genesis, as Sarah and Abraham wait impatiently into their nineties before God grants them a son. Think of what God said to Abraham: "And I will make thy seed as the dust of the earth: so that if a man can number the dust of the earth, then shall thy seed also be numbered."

From that penis springs the fulfillment of God's promise. Sex drives the biblical narrative. That is why Abraham makes his servant place his hand on his penis to swear. Sex bears the word and the power of God himself. And for that reason it is to be understood as the most sacred of human activities. It is not enough for Abraham's son to ejaculate, to copulate, to reproduce. He must do so in the right way. He must circumcise the organ. He must marry a woman who can live up to the promise. And so, likewise, we must learn to respect the awesome significance of the sexual act by following the strictures and rituals the Torah gives us to sacralize it, or at least by meditating upon their meaning. That goes not just for circumcision, which, of course, has made itself palatable to the modern mind by passing for hygiene, but also for the more troubling edicts, such as the rules about when a wife is impure to her husband.

I remember noting, at the time, that Rabbi Paul gave us an out. We could *meditate* on the laws. We didn't always have to follow them. I didn't entirely agree with him about that. It struck me as arbitrary. How do you decide which laws to follow and which ones to meditate on? Nor did he, who was so strict about some things and not so strict about others, always agree with himself. He manifested all the contradictoriness of the American Conservative movement, to which he tenaciously adhered; the effort to juggle modernity and the ancient mechanisms of rabbinic law produced many contortions, such as permission to drive a car on the Sabbath. Rabbi Paul was always able to cite some well-thought-through Conservative ruling to justify some apparent Conservative oxymoron, and, of course, I was not qualified to judge the merits of those. But his apparent contradictoriness made me love him with a protective tenderness that was all the more fierce and tender because he had made himself so offensive to everyone else.

I took, I have to admit, a rather adolescent pleasure in playing the rabbi's defender during the many synagogue social events at which his flaws were anatomized and deplored. But I genuinely loved the man. I loved his arrogance, his abruptness, his bullheadedness. His difficultness embodied, for me, the difficultness of religion itself. If he was hapless, religion was hapless. At least he wasn't a smooth talker effacing its unpleasantnesses with a free application of smarm, which had previously been my idea of what religious professionals do.

I loved him because he showed me how to love Jewish law. I knew (though I often pretended to myself that I didn't know) that I would never be born again as an Orthodox Jew. I would never, for example, observe the laws of *niddah,* which determine at which point in a woman's menstrual cycle she may have sex with her husband. Nor would I be able to uproot myself and join the kind of community that would make it possible for me to follow every jot and tittle of Sabbath law. But I could also refuse to reject such laws as merely antiquated. I could allow myself to love them. I could hold them in my mind as if they were poems to live by. For though I knew that blood is life, when it pours out of my body, I could remember the laws of *niddah* and know that blood is also death, which is why one is supposed to purify oneself after menstruation. I could remember that menstruation is also a tragedy, albeit on a very small scale—the disappearance of a possible life, the evanescence of an angelic ghost—and soon to be overturned by the joyous comedy of ovulation. I didn't want a baby when I first had this thought. But *niddah* is what first made me grasp the enormity of the fact that I *could* have one. And as with *niddah,* so with the Sabbath. I need not *be* a Sabbatarian to be a Sabbatarian. I could grasp, even celebrate, the urgent necessity of a day of rest without cutting myself off from the busy, convenient, 24/7 world that I knew and loved.

Or could I?

PART SEVEN

REMEMBERING THE SABBATH

1.

CAN WE DO NOTHING MORE THAN TURN THE SABBATH OVER IN OUR minds, the way we would a poem, and extract from it anything worth having?

The answer is obvious: obviously yes, and obviously no. Of course the Sabbath is worth mulling over—everything is—and of course you can't derive much lasting benefit from a regularly observed period of rest if you don't observe it regularly. Even if you do nothing but re-member the Sabbath, though, you press your nose up against a differ-ent order of time, and that has its uses. For one thing, it will make you appreciate the near-impossibility of bringing it back. We have changed too much to contemplate its return, at least in its old form, even though the bulk of that change has happened in a short span of time.

As recently as at the beginning of the past century—to revert to that great lurch toward modernity—Sunday mornings in the United States were still filled "with Sunday school [and] church," as the American historian Alexis McCrossen writes, as well as "excursions, picnics, movies, and trolley rides." In 1908, G. Stanley Hall, the psychologist and, most famously, the Clark University president who invited Sigmund Freud to visit America, eulogized Sunday's domestic charms: "freedom from all slavery to the clock, better and more leisurely toilets and meals, the hush of noise on the deserted street, the greatly intensified charm of the sky, sunshine, trees, fields, pleasant morning anticipations for the day, more zest for reading and perhaps study, converse with friends, calls, visits, correspondence, as well as rest pure and simple, for body and mind."

Hall's lovely essay, however, laid bare the contradiction that doomed his high-minded Sabbatarianism. Hall, a churchgoing Protestant and a man of practical bent, begged Americans to adopt "the scientific Sunday"—the psychologically and physically hygienic day that Dickens pressed for, a day of exercise, highbrow entertainment, and family "walks and talks and nature lessons." Innocent and appealing as this "scientific" Sunday sounds, it spelled the end of the Sabbatarian Sunday.

Before we can understand why, though, we have to remember the kind of Sabbath Hall was reacting to. In 1908, strict Sunday-closing laws remained in force in seventeen states and in Indian territory. They banned amusements, fishing, and hunting, as well as selling and working. Hall's own Sunday had a milder rigor to it, but a rigor nonetheless. In his home state of Massachusetts, he had the right to buy a Sunday paper, that amalgam of news and gossip and fashion advice that Sabbatarian ministers still railed against. He could smoke a pipe; Massachusetts did not forbid the sale of tobacco. By comparison, many of the western states, which passed their Sunday-closing laws just as the old-time behavioral codes had begun to lose their force, were far more permissive. In Wyoming, as Hall points out, he could send a telegraph, repair farm equipment, smelt metal and glass, and buy ice cream, milk, fresh meat, and bread. In New Mexico, he could conduct business as usual on Sunday; only the kinds of work and amusements that might disturb congregations and families were prohibited.

Hall applauded this latter sort of active and permissive Sabbath, as long as it preserved a Christian decorum. Let "mild drinks" be served,

so that "gross intoxication" would not be sought. Let there be innocent entertainments at which the sexes could commingle, so that vice
would not be indulged in. Let children out of doors to play sports and
games, and let adults play their sports and games, too. America had to
make Sunday a day of leisure, Hall argued, if it was to have a Sunday
at all.

Not that such changes weren't already under way. In the previous
half century, museums, libraries, and world's fairs had all begun opening on Sundays, along with movie theaters and baseball stadiums. And
those places were where the contradictions between the "scientific"
and the "Sabbatarian" Sunday became unavoidable. The problem
with substituting cultural consumption and active leisure for rest is
that one person's recreation is another person's work. If museums, libraries, and baseball stadiums are to stay open, then security guards
and librarians have to work, and baseball players have to play.

Legislators tried to keep pace with changing mores by expanding
the scope of "works of necessity and charity"; that is, the work required for the maintenance of expected standards of living and the
enjoyment of leisure. Utilities were to keep providing power and
water on Sundays; deliverymen were to keep depositing ice and milk
at front doors. Presses kept printing, operators kept connecting telephone calls, radio and television stations kept broadcasting. Amusement parks, national parks, opera houses, restaurants, cigar stores, train
stations, and airports kept serving up all the other goods and services
required by their customers and patrons.

What destroyed the reign of blue laws, though, wasn't just that
everyone went to work on Sunday—the Sunday service sector remained relatively small in proportion to the rest of the economy—but
also that the definition of "necessity and charity" broadened until the
line it drew between life and work began to seem laughable. The distinctions between permissible and non-permissible Sunday commerce had always varied from state to state and county to county, but
the laws had evinced a rough consensus of what was proper on Sunday and what wasn't. By the middle of the twentieth century, though,
you could dine at a restaurant in one city but not in another. Even if

you stayed within city lines, you could buy an item in one neighborhood but not in another, or you could buy *this* item at a store but not
that one at the same store. Tackle shops and beach burger shacks
stayed open; downtown department stores didn't. You could buy film
from a photo shop on the boardwalk, but not the camera needed to
use it.

Sunday-closing laws came under attack in the courts for failing to
pass what is called a "rational basis test." They discriminated so un-
predictably among activities, varied so widely from one region to
another, and were enforced so randomly that they violated the due-
process clause of the Fourteenth Amendment, which guarantees
equal protection to all citizens. The other criticism that emerged was
that Sunday-closing laws violated the First Amendment, which forbids the establishment of a particular religion and endorses freedom of
religious practice. Religious minorities, such as Seventh-Day Adventists and Orthodox Jews, began to file lawsuits objecting to having to
close their stores for two days of the week, Saturday and Sunday. In response to those challenges, several states began to make exceptions for
Saturday Sabbath-keepers.

The Supreme Court's decision in *McGowan et al. v. Maryland*
(1961) upheld Sunday-closing laws on the grounds that the government's interest in the well-being of the majority of its citizens over-
rode whatever burdens Sunday laws imposed on the minority. Justice
Felix Frankfurter, recognizing that to the unsympathetic eye the laws
looked like what one skeptic later called a "gallimaufry," or potpourri,
insisted that they were not irrational. It was possible to draw a
"reasonable line of demarcation" between those activities that "add
enjoyment" to Sunday and those that needlessly deprive employees of
their day.

But the sense of urgency that held that line of demarcation was
ebbing away. McCrossen points out that the success of the labor
movement also helped dim Sunday's luster. In the earlier decades of
the twentieth century, activists agitating for shorter hours—with occasional though unreliable support from Sunday Sabbatarian organizations—had managed to shorten the workweek to five days from six

or seven, and the workday to eight hours from ten or twelve. The first five-day workweek was granted in 1908 at a New England mill that employed many Jewish workers. Henry Ford was the first major manufacturer to adopt the five-day week; he grasped that the American people needed more time to shop if they were going to buy his cars. In 1938, the Fair Labor Standards Act established the forty-hour workweek and eight-hour day as the norm and gave the ordinary working person so many more free hours that the labor-free Sunday seemed less urgent than before.

The group that really turned Sunday inside out, though, was women. As they poured into the workforce in the 1960s and the 1970s, they had less time to shop during the week. More of women's traditional domestic duties—cooking, cleaning, child care—had to be outsourced. Divorce became more common, and with it single parents, male as well as female, who had no choice but to shop on weekends.

Businesses quickly perceived the demand for Sunday shopping hours and began lobbying state legislatures to make those hours legal. Not all businesses supported repeal of the Sunday laws. Some department-store owners actually preferred the old way of doing things, in some cases out of personal religious conviction and in some cases because they doubted that opening on Sunday would actually increase sales, rather than spread the same quantity of sales over seven days instead of six. Many small businesses resisted opening on Sunday, too, fearing that the cost of Sunday labor—proportionally greater for them than for larger establishments—would make it harder for them to compete. Some small businesses enjoyed special exemptions that allowed them to stay open on Sunday (which businesses qualified for exemptions varied state by state); these gave mom-and-pop stores an extra weapon in their arsenal in the battle to ward off the chain stores, so they had no interest in changing the status quo.

It was the chain stores that worked hardest to persuade legislatures to do away with Sunday laws. Some states abolished their blue laws only after campaigns organized and funded by chain retailers, such as Kmart, Toys "R" Us, Sears, Walgreens, Bradlees, Stop & Shop, and

Home Depot. And while the enemies of blue laws acted in their own self-interest, they also made an argument that was designed to appeal to politicians and their constituents. By dampening competition, they said, Sunday restrictions kept retail prices artificially high. Protecting small businesses may have been good public policy, but, the bigger businesses argued, it was bad economics. States that repealed the laws would be able to cut prices, attract new businesses, and create jobs.

In 1961, when *McGowan et al. v. Maryland* was handed down, forty-nine states outlawed something on Sunday that was legal the other six days of the week, even if the forbidden activity was nothing more threatening to the Sunday peace than barbering or the sale of liquor. (Alaska was the only state that had no blue laws at the time.) Today, a majority of states have such laws on the books, but they do little to preserve Frankfurter's "atmosphere of entire community repose," nor do they back up his claim that the line of demarcation between permissible and non-permissible activities is "reasonable." These days, no two sets of blue laws look remotely alike; each is riddled with oddly specific proscriptions and exceptions; all are laxly or inconsistently enforced; and very few people even know they exist.

The most common blue laws restrict sales of alcohol on some period on Sunday, usually the morning. But there is indeed a potpourri of other proscriptions. Arkansas, Illinois, Louisiana, Maryland, Maine, and New Hampshire outlaw Sunday horse racing. Maine enjoins boxing, air circuses, and wrestling. Arkansas disallows Sunday dog racing. Connecticut and Tennessee forbid Sunday car racing. Connecticut, Maryland, New Jersey, and North Carolina impose complicated and highly qualified restrictions on Sunday hunting. New Jersey and Virginia forbid oyster fishing on Sunday. Baltimore County, in Maryland, prohibits bingo on Sunday, while New Jersey bans all Sunday "games of chance." Tennessee requires that all "adult" establishments shut down for the day. Several states shut down car showrooms on Sunday, although that particular prohibition has been singled out for attack in recent years and is fast disappearing.

To make matters more confusing, many states allow cities and counties to opt out of the blue laws if they want to. A large number do, or make exceptions for kinds of labor or business that happen to be important to their economies. For instance, South Carolina bans "worldly work . . . and business" but exempts rubber and plastic mold-making, as well as textile manufacturing. New Jersey allows munici-palities to opt *in* to its blue laws; naturally, few do. (Paramus, which lies right across the Hudson River from New York City and has a high concentration of big-box stores, is one borough that has opted in, a fact that occasions bitter complaints from New Yorkers looking for weekend access to cheaper merchandise.)

It can be argued (and has been argued) that Sunday-closing laws reflect the interventions of so many special interests that they can no longer protect the communal aspect of the day of rest. One legal scholar goes further, declaring that since many of the laws that remain prohibit not work but recreational activities such as gambling and hunting, they can be interpreted only as fossils from America's theo-cratic days and should be ruled unconstitutional.

2.

IT'S TRUE. The Sabbath *is* a fossil. It's the past hardened into rock, whereas time becomes more fluid with each passing day. Cell-phone and text-messaging and social-networking technologies have begun to wash away at adamantine "mechanical time," the unyielding time of clocks, and to suspend us within "mobile time," which can be made to flow whichever way we want. Whereas what is called Universal Time emanates from an atomic clock at the Royal Observatory in Greenwich, England, the time of mobile communications emanates from each of us individually. Universal Time coordinates local time around the globe, so that institutions and the public know when to interact with one another. Using our cell phones and other devices, we micro-coordinate our time with that of our associates, which al-lows us to bypass Universal Time and operate on what I would call Particular Time—time that can constantly be adjusted to fit our own idiosyncratic needs. If we encounter traffic jams on our way to a ren-dezvous, we can call or text and prepare our friends or colleagues for late arrivals. If six college friends don't know enough about their schedules in the morning to make a plan for the evening, they can simply communicate with one another electronically over the course of the next several hours until they arrive at one. "The mobile telephone relaxes the implicit contracts around time," the sociologist Richard Ling writes. "It softens the schedule."

As we grow accustomed to ever softer time contracts, the Sabbath's granitic temporality begins to seem ever more unreasonable. Very few situations require fanatical punctuality anymore. Moreover, a softer schedule uses time more efficiently. No longer need we squander precious minutes waiting for dates who don't show up, or on other scheduling mishaps (although it should be said that we lose some of that saved time in making and refining our plans). As a result, accommodating ourselves to the uncompromising demands of the Sabbath schedule becomes less a matter of fitting it into our calendars than of forcing ourselves to conform to a kind of time that seems obsolete. Remembering and keeping the Sabbath under these conditions also exact a higher social price. More friends and colleagues lift a querying eyebrow when we say that we can't be reached or disturbed for a full twenty-five hours than were likely to have done so in the days before phone calls and emails could track us down at any location. In short, the advent of mobile time erodes the plausibility of the Sabbath the way coastal waters turn boulders into sand.

This sea change isn't as complete as it may yet become. The large temporal frameworks of our lives remain fairly firm. We still work comparatively standard hours or go to school from morning till afternoon, fall through spring. But to the degree that electronics take over our activities and our interactions, personal time becomes more fungible. We shop when it's convenient, not when stores are open. We watch movies and television on DVDs and On Demand and TiVo, not according to published schedules. We correspond via email and Twitter and Facebook in instant, staccato bursts throughout the day, or over the course of several days, not when the mail is delivered.

Mobile time is time that *we're* in charge of, and who would want to lose that? Ling says that he has found a "gendered dimension" to the way people talk about this kind of time in interviews. Temporal flexibility finds its most passionate advocates among those with the sharpest conflicts between personal time and public time, which is to say working mothers (although this description also fits working care-givers of all kinds). These women often find themselves coordinating the loose, task-oriented time of child rearing and home maintenance with the closely measured, more fixed time of the workplace. Moth-ers today can call babysitters at any hour, be reached anywhere in case of emergency, be asked to pick up milk or antibiotic ointment and Band-Aids on their way home even if they've already left the office. All this allows them to manage their complicated lives with an ease their mothers would never have dreamed of.

But being in perpetual contact can also make us feel as if time is in charge of us. In that case, we may be experiencing what sociologists call the Lazarus effect, the nagging consciousness of "dead" time that wouldn't strike us as wasted if we didn't have a mobile device in our hands. Micro-coordination, being more efficient, also sets a more ex-acting standard of time use. It used to be possible to wiggle free of the Lazarus effect by taking yourself off the grid, but that option is fast vanishing. Five years ago, when I went on summer vacation, I could tell my friends and colleagues that it might be days before I could log on and get their messages because the impoverished Catskill Moun-tain town where I rented a house hadn't yet been wired for broad-band. Now that the region has entered the twenty-first century, that excuse no longer works.

We might, if we were inventive grammarians, call this state of being incessantly *on* the "embryonic progressive tense." "Progressive" in the grammatical sense—in the progressive tense we don't complete an action, we are in the process of doing it—because we are available and attached to others on a continuing basis, not just in the present but also in the past, and in all likelihood in the future, too. And "em-bryonic" because cell phones function like umbilical cords, tethering friends and family who might otherwise drift off and become artifacts of our personal histories, and because social-network sites fish out of oblivion the high-school classmates, office co-workers, and one-night stands who would otherwise vanish without a trace. In the embryonic progressive, nothing ends. The Sabbath, by contrast, demands of us a hard and tragic sense of beginnings and ends.

3.
———

WHEN AND IF THE SABBATH GOES, here are the forms of time that might go, too: non-instrumental time, bounded time, shared time, and rhythmic time. We need non-instrumental time to remember our "human condition," as Arendt put it; we need bounded and shared time to become a society; and we need rhythmic time to make the previous three a habit. But two questions remain. First, hasn't our enhanced connectedness made it unnecessary to set aside time to be together? And, second, are habits really all that great?

Electronic communications may turn out to increase the frequency of real-world contacts, rather than replace them. After all, our heightened ability to synchronize our schedules has made it easier to get together. So maybe we have all the community we can handle, and what we want is to be alone! Besides, mobile communication liberates us. It alleviates the burdens of self-presentation. It's a lot easier to be ourselves typing at home in our underwear than talking face-to-face.

There is one big difference, though, between face-to-face and electronic interlocution. That is what psychologists call "co-presence," which provides, they say, "attunement." The value of physical togetherness lies in the possibility of aligning ourselves to others at the deepest physical level. Tests have shown that people laughing together soon begin to gasp and whoop to the same convulsive beat. People happily talking together mirror one another's blinks, nods, and finger taps. Electroencephalograph (EEG) recordings of the brains of infants and adults exchanging coos show that their brain waves rise and fall at the same time. "Face-to-face social interaction takes place among physiological systems, not merely among individuals as cognitive systems or bodily actors," the sociologist Randall Collins writes. "From an evolutionary perspective, it is not surprising that human beings, like other animals, are neurologically wired to respond to each other; and social situations that call forth these responses are experienced as highly rewarding."

Perhaps we have begun to forget why being together feels good. Being shy myself, I'd almost always rather type than talk. Or maybe the pleasure of owning a cool gadget is greater than the pleasures described above. Still possessed of an old-fashioned clamshell cell phone, I certainly have iPhone envy. In any case, we are witnessing a decline in the status of the physical. A tellingly coarse term has emerged to describe real-time and real-space encounters: "flesh meets." I once watched a young rabbi sitting next to me at a seminar-sized meeting furtively tapping on his BlackBerry under the lip of the table, even as the courtly elderly director of a major Jewish charity went around the room introducing one person to another. The fact that even a rabbi felt entitled to withdraw his fullest attention from the events in the room during the performance of such an important social ritual said, I thought, everything.

Is it possible to imagine what might happen to, say, family or community life without the regular—that is, habitual and scheduled—coordination of our physiological systems? Yes, because we have seen what happens when a society dispenses altogether with the common calendar that makes this possible. In 1929, one year into the Soviet Union's First Five-Year Plan to speed up industrialization, the Council of People's Commissars adopted the continuous workweek, the *nepreryvka,* so that no production facility need ever lie idle. The idea was to divide the working population into subgroups and stagger each group's day of rest. At the same time, the Council reduced the week from seven days to five by eliminating Saturday and Sunday. This was probably meant as an attack on religion, since both days were tainted by their association with the religious calendar.

Eviatar Zerubavel tells the story in *The Seven Day Circle*. He writes: "The Soviet authorities essentially divided the entire society into five separate populations, staggered vis-à-vis one another like the different voices in a polyphonic, five-voice fugue." On any given day, 80 percent of the labor force would be at work and 20 percent at home—but not necessarily with the rest of their families. By then many Soviet women worked, and no effort was made to coordinate their schedules with those of their husbands and children. The reformers may even have meant to break up families, since according to Marxist ideology the family was irredeemably bourgeois. But your *nepreryvka* worker on his or her day off was hard-pressed to come up with company. Clubs, shows, and even (God forbid) churches struggled to stay open, since none of them could attract much attendance on any given day. Workers' meetings puttered to a halt. Bored and lonely, Soviet workers had no choice but to socialize with people who were on the same schedule. Each day was given its own color—the "first day" was yellow, the "second day" was peach, and so on. Zerubavel reports that people began categorizing one another in their address books according to their color.

What made the continuous workweek a flop from Stalin's point of view, though, was that it slowed production. Workers resented the strain on family life. They didn't like the new schedule's effect on the workplace, either. To deal with workers' absences every fifth day, managers had to move people around, assigning them to fill in on this task, then that one. Workers felt cut off from their jobs, their machines, their co-workers—from everything that had previously given them pride and pleasure in their work. In June of 1931, Stalin gave a speech in which he said that, as a result of the *nepreryvka,* "we have the lack of any sense of responsibility, careless handling of machines, mass breakage, and the absence of an incentive to increase the productivity of labor." Five months later, the Council discontinued the continuous workweek, although it waited nine more years to reinstate the seven-day week.

The *nepreryvka* didn't just disrupt family life; it disrupted long-standing patterns of work and rest, which, when shared by the general society, are usually called customs. So are customs per se worth preserving? Certainly a long line of philosophers and psychologists have thought so. Customs, as David Hume famously said, are "the great guide of human life." William James called habit—by which he meant both habits and customs—"the enormous flywheel of society, its most precious conservative agent." In his book *The Metronomic Society* (1988), the sociologist Michael Young speculated that humans are genetically programmed to turn memories into customs, since they're such unimpeachable devices of social self-replication.

We don't generally see habits as assets. The word *habit* usually invokes behaviors that we would rather get rid of. Habits are mindless, obsessive, animal-like. We are *creatures* of habit; we'd rather be masters of our fate.

James, however, argued that habit is both necessary and efficient—it reduces unnecessary expenditures of physical and intellectual energy and facilitates higher-level thinking. In *The Principles of Psychology,* he quotes an eloquent Dr. Carpenter on the subject: "When we are learning to walk, to ride, to swim, skate, fence, write, play, or sing, we interrupt ourselves at every step by unnecessary movements and false notes. When we are proficient, on the contrary, the results not only follow with the very minimum of muscular action requisite to bring them forth, they also follow from a single instantaneous 'cue.' The marksman sees the bird, and, before he knows it, he has aimed and shot." A pilot whose flying skills hadn't become instinctive would have had less attention to devote to saving his plane when a flock of birds struck his engines. Businesses that don't standardize their procedures to the point where they become a part of institutional second nature would never be able to coordinate their production processes.

It is true that habit is unconscious. Brain scans of people acting out of habit show that the mental correlate of the activity bypasses the prefrontal cortex, which houses consciousness as well as explicit memories. Instead, habits light up the subcortical structures of the brain, the cerebellum and the basal ganglia, where we store implicit or subconscious memories. Habits even change the shape of the brain. The biologist Eric R. Kandel reports that, nearly half a century ago, he and other neuroscientists discovered that habituation in animals—conditioning that makes them respond automatically to a stimulus—alters the connections between their synapses.

Teachers understand the power of habit; that's why they stress good study habits. Parents and bosses do, too. They also know that the best way to get you to agree to do something is to get you to do it. Since habits defy the belief that our wills should be sovereign, we tell ourselves that we *meant* to do things that way. Max Weber elevates this psychological trick to a sociological dictum: "The mere fact of regular recurrence of certain events somehow confers on them the dignity of oughtness."

Recent experiments by psychologists have demonstrated that we're likely to categorize something as true simply because we've heard it before, rather than because we have good reason to believe it to be true. The psychologist Christian Unkelbach, having conducted one such test, speculates that familiar statements are easier to process, and that we mistake this ease for truth: "Processing fluency," says Unkelbach, creates a "truth-effect."

On the other hand, just because something has a "truth-effect" doesn't mean that it isn't true. Familiarity *is* a likely indicator of truth. A statement may be true in only one way, but it can be wrong in a million different ways. The earth is round, not flat or cylindrical or bolus-shaped. We tend to hear true statements more often than false ones.

P, the priestly writer of the Bible and the codifier of Sabbath law, also had a deep—you might say neurotheological—grasp of how habits and customs work on the mind. There is a curious moment in Exodus when Moses reads the laws to the Israelites gathered at Mount Sinai and the Israelites respond, *Na'aseh v'nishma*—"We do and we hear." The verbs, as commentators have pointed out, are in the wrong order. Shouldn't the people have *heard* before they agreed to *do*? But it is in the doing that we hear what a ritual, or a law, or a custom, has come to tell us, and in the doing that we begin to believe it to be the right thing to do.

4.
—

THE UTILITARIAN ARGUMENT for remembering the Sabbath, then, would be that it reminds us to get in the habit of not working and spending quality time with the people around us. Doing that—and thereby coming to believe that it was the right thing to do—would benefit us, our families, our neighborhoods, and our nation, nurturing all the informal and formal associations that go into the making of our civil society.

Another argument for remembering the Sabbath is less hygienic; it appeals instead to what Presidents Lincoln and Obama have called the better angels of our nature. This is Wordsworth's spot in time in which we cultivate our negative capabilities. I should say that this argument is only rarely advanced in the name of the Sabbath. It more often takes the form of a lament for the lost art of leisure, as elevated to its highest form by the ancient Greeks and Romans. In 1948, as Germany grimly set about to rebuild its shattered economy, the German Catholic philosopher Josef Pieper wrote a book on leisure in which he begged his readers not to succumb to the ethos of "total work" and forget the ancient understanding of leisure as the highest good, the point of life, that which makes possible the highest achievements of the human spirit, philosophy and music. "Leisure," wrote Pieper, "is a form of silence, of that silence which is the prerequisite of the apprehension of reality." In 1962, the American political philosopher Sebastian de Grazia defended leisure in the name of Aristotle, who thought that a citizen could not be free without leisure and the ability to use it well.

More recently, David Levy, a professor at the Information School at the University of Washington, has updated both the utilitarian and the humanistic arguments for the networked age by calling for a new "informational environmentalism." Just as we fight to save marshlands and old-growth forests from development and pollution, he says, so we need to fight to save ourselves from the "pollutants" of communications overload: the overabundance of information that turns us into triagers and managers, rather than readers; the proliferation of bad or useless or ersatz information; the forces that push us to process information quickly rather than thoughtfully. If we don't fend off those pollutants, he cautions, we risk becoming cut off from the world, rather than more connected; less able to make wise decisions, rather than better informed; and, in the end, less human. "Much as the modern-day environmental movement has worked to cultivate and preserve certain natural habitats, such as wetlands and old-growth forests, for the health of the planet, so too should we now begin to cultivate and preserve human habitats for the sake of our own well-being," Levy writes.

How would we go about this? Levy models his answer, he says, on the environmentalist movement. Just as environmentalists no longer try to shut down factories or get rid of cities, information environmentalists should not try to slow down the pace of life or limit the information revolution. Instead, he says, "we will need to cultivate unhurried activities and quiet places, sanctuaries in time and space for reflection and contemplation." Which sanctuary in time does he have in mind? The Sabbath, of course. "I by no means want to argue for the broad-scale adoption of traditional Sabbath practices . . . by the larger population," he says. What does he want to argue for? He is loath to say: "I could speak to the ways I myself am experimenting with such ideas at home and in the workplace, but effective change will most importantly come through collective reflection, experimentation, and action: local communities creating sanctuaries that fit their particular circumstances."

5.

So what if, having remembered the Sabbath, we *did* want to bring it back? What aspect would we find desirable? How would we go about doing something so eccentric and retrograde?

We have, it seems to me, two options. We could bring it back individually or we could bring it back collectively. Cultivating a Sabbath habit one person at a time has an obvious appeal. Every good Jewish missionary—that is, a person whose job is to lure Jews back into the fold—knows that it is best to start one's evangelizing by preaching the virtues of Shabbat. Chabad houses, run by a Hasidic group from Brooklyn known as the Lubavitchers, send forth battalions of young black-hatted Jews to invite college students and lonely Jewish travelers to celebrate Shabbat in Lubavitch homes around the world. At the Orthodox synagogue that I sometimes visit with my husband on Friday nights, men vie with one another to invite us to their homes, where their wives have cooked elaborate meals. Reform and Conservative congregations launch campaigns to increase Saturday attendance that have names like "Celebrate Shabbat" or "Shabbat Club."

Classical Jewish theology presents the Sabbath as a communal good, rather than an individual one, but communitarianism can be a hard sell in a land of rugged individuals. When the anthropologist Riv-Ellen Prell studied some of these synagogue programs, she found that congregants responded most enthusiastically to pitches that emphasized personal well-being. Celebrating Shabbat met their need for "relaxation and self-reflection . . . family . . . a break from busy-ness, technology, consumerism, and modernity."

Christian Sabbatarianism has also begun to make a comeback, stressing the psychological benefits to the individual rather than the rightness of obeying God. A strictly unscientific survey on Amazon.com turned up more than twenty guides to bringing the Sabbath back into your life, all published in the past decade. To the degree that Christianity enters into the discussion at all, it is seen as a tool of self-improvement. And a secular Sabbath has emerged that is largely a way of curing an addiction to technology. Adherents to what's called a "technology Sabbath"—naturally, they stay in touch via the Internet—speak of themselves in language that evokes Alcoholics Anonymous testimonials: "I love technology. I'm not a Luddite. But I realized it was a problem when I would sit down to check my e-mail and it was almost like I would wake up six hours later and find I was watching videos of puppies on YouTube," Ariel Meadow Stallings, a blogger from Seattle, told the Reuters news agency in April 2008. "I'd try and think what I had been doing for the past two hours and I had no idea. I associate that kind of time loss with blackouts when you're drunk."

In its celebration of self-discipline, secular Sabbatarianism has a surface resemblance to the Orthodox and Puritan Sabbaths, but it has

a deeper affinity to other, recent movements in which Americans take
themselves off the grid: the voluntary simplicity movement, the green
or sustainability movement, the frugality movement. There are rules
to these movements, and you are urged to keep them; the voluntary
simplicity movement, for instance, discourages eating out and eating
high on the food chain (meat) and unnecessary consumption. But in
the end you are accountable to no one but yourself. You have the
good of society in mind but all you can expect to change is your own
behavior, and maybe that of a few people around you.

The philosopher Michel Foucault had a name for such personal
quests for transformation: He called them techniques of the self. He
did not mean to be derogatory. In the third volume of *The History of
Sexuality: The Care of the Self,* Foucault locates the origins of the technique of the self in the writings of the ancients—Seneca and Marcus
Aurelius and Plutarch and Epictetus. These philosophers sought,
among other things, to achieve sexual moderation in cultures rife
with promiscuity. They shared "a mistrust of the pleasures, an emphasis on the consequences of their abuse for the body and the soul, a val-
orization of marriage and marital obligations, a disaffection with
regard to the spiritual meanings imputed to the love of boys," Foucault wrote. This was not a puritanical backlash, exactly; it was more
like applied philosophy. Plato, too, stressed "taking care of oneself." In
the Socratic dialogues with the young future statesman and general
Alcibiades—who apparently had a wild streak—Socrates scolds him
for wanting to take charge of Athens when he has not learned to govern himself. He had yet to learn, said Socrates, the *techne tou biou,* "the
art of existence."

An appealing feature of the technique of the self is that it is voluntary. There is no talk of legislating morality. Nor is the regimen
meant for everybody. On the contrary, being able to stick to the rules
is what distinguished the adept from the throng. This austere self-
discipline became the basis, in part, of Christian monasticism; it
seeped into rabbinic thought. The Greeks and the Romans attained
transcendence through determined moderation; monks, saints, and

mystics by giving up the pleasures of the flesh; and the great rabbinic sages by performing heroic feats of Torah study and demonstrating piety above and beyond the Law.

Today's neo-Sabbatarians, in other words, are the latest in a long line of philosophical and spiritual élites. They give things up in a spirit of protest or in an effort to bring holiness into their lives. But their reforms play out in very limited spheres, often on the margins of society. People suffering from time deprivation or information overload may not be addicted or driven or out of touch with the higher purpose of life. They may be tied to their meetings and computers against their will—by the need to hold on to a job. Individualized Sabbatarianism may change life for the lucky few, but it won't help the many.

6.

THE OTHER WAY to bring back the Sabbath would be to re-regulate, collectively, the use of our time. Do I mean mean bringing back blue laws? These happen to be underrated, in my opinion. However complicated, unsystematic, and occasionally unjust they may have been, they did succeed in staving off the encroachments of the market and the specter of 24/7 labor—Stalin's continuous workweek—for quite a long time.

But restricting Sunday commerce makes no sense anymore. For one thing, it places the burden on the people who can least afford to carry it—the women, usually, who are already juggling children, households, and full-time jobs. For another, it's nonsensical to proscribe activities, such as the purchase of alcohol, that nobody frowns on anymore, especially if everything else is for sale. In any case, it is no longer possible to draw a "reasonable line of demarcation" between shopping and recreation, since shopping has evolved into a kind of entertainment and entertainment has largely devolved into a series of long-form commercials for worldwide celebrity brands.

The emphasis on commerce seems misplaced, anyway. The Fourth Commandment doesn't explicitly forbid us to shop. It tells us not to work, and not to force others to work. Now, no modern society, no matter how Sabbatarian—Israel is a good example—can avoid putting some people to work on the Sabbath. Any high-functioning state needs uninterrupted access to hospitals, drugstores, the military, food, water, transportation, and other basic services; indeed, Israel makes all those things available to its citizens on Saturday. Any society with a large secular population will also require a full panoply of recreational and self-care options on its days off, including, I would argue, retail shopping. Israel has plenty of that, too, although owing to inconsistent enforcement of its Sabbath laws it is not entirely clear how much Saturday commerce and labor is legal and how much simply flouts the laws.

Nor does the Fourth Commandment tell us not to work too hard, or too long. Indeed, as the Puritans stressed, we're *supposed* to work the other six days. The Fourth Commandment tells us to remember to (1) stop working, (2) stop working at the same time, and (3) stop working at regular intervals. The implication is that a society has a right, and perhaps an obligation, to marshal its temporal resources for the benefit of the greatest number, even at the risk of harming the few.

The United States, in the twenty-first century, happens to be particularly oblivious to this particular Bible lesson. We have remarkably few laws governing the use and abuse of workers' time. Two out of three countries in the world have laws that dictate the maximum number of hours employees can be expected to work (usually between forty-eight and sixty hours a week). The United States is not among them. Employees in most countries are entitled to rest breaks, but American employees are not. America has fewer public holidays than most industrialized nations. American workers have no legal right to take a vacation; vacation policy is determined by the employer. Most European countries require employers to give workers three to six weeks of paid vacation.

America does, of course, have the Fair Labor Standards Act. Adopted at the height of the Great Depression, the FLSA was passed less to protect workers than to fix a broken economy: It was meant to redistribute employment from the few who had it and who worked long hours (the average workweek was forty-eight hours), to include the many who were out of a job. The history of the FLSA, it should be said, tells a cautionary tale about the unintended consequences of regulating time, for it appears to have fostered the current climate of overwork. In the 1950s, the era of the organization man, working overtime at time and a half became a way to climb from the lower-middle class to the middle-middle class, as well as the obligatory proof of one's seriousness about one's job. Because the FLSA exempted executive, administrative, and professional employees (in addition to farmworkers, whose work was assumed to require long hours), it wound up contributing to "the time divide"—the gap in American society between high-earning salaried élites who either drive themselves or are pressured into working much longer than forty hours, and, on the other hand, low-earning workers whose hours are deliberately kept below forty hours a week. Some of these workers may put in more than forty hours, but only by combining part-time jobs. As a result, they don't get overtime—or health benefits, either.

In any case, a lot has changed since the FLSA was passed. For one thing, in 1938 it was assumed that the forty hours of the workweek would be allocated in even chunks across five days (Monday through Friday). That assumption can no longer be made. Another assumption underlying the forty-hour week is that it represented forty hours of paid work per household, with the same amount of time or more being devoted, usually by a wife, to all the essential unpaid duties. The rise of dual-earning couples, with the increase in single-parent families, means that each household has less time to devote to those activities. The loss of non-work time in these families has made it harder for them to cope with the needs of family members on different schedules, such as schoolchildren and elderly parents; that is why workers are asking for, and receiving, flextime.

This steady stream of small adjustments to the common work schedule is another way in which we are edging closer to Pieper's specter of "total work." When American courts and labor arbitrators hear "disputes at the boundaries of time," as the law professor Todd Rakoff calls them—that is, tugs-of-war between workers and management over the proper use of workers' time—their decisions tend to favor companies over individuals, the time of the organizations over the time of families. For instance, a worker who refuses to work overtime has very little legal protection against being fired or disciplined for doing so; the right to refuse overtime is negotiated contract by contract, usually by unions, except in the case of government workers, who enjoy the protections of civil-service law. When an employee *is* fired or disciplined for refusing to work overtime because he or she needed to pick up a child from school or day care—a situation that generates its fair share of labor disputes—judges and arbitrators have generally held that the worker was required to make a "reasonable" effort to come up with some other arrangement before saying no. One such decision featured a carpenter who walked out on a job where he was working overtime because he had to pick up his two young children from a day-care center that was about to close. The arbitrator ruled that he should have left the children at the day-care center. He didn't need to leave just then, because he knew that the day-care center would have taken care of the children for an extra fee.

Rakoff suggests three possible reasons for the law's reluctance to protect non-work time. One is the imbalance of power between workers and management. Another is the outmoded assumption that workers have someone at home who can take care of such things. Both reasons seem true but remediable. Rakoff's third explanation lays the blame on a more intractable, because more elusive, condition: "cultural blindness" about time. That is, we have a hard time seeing non-work time as anything but formless leisure, rather than time spent doing things that have to be done if society is to thrive, and done regularly and collectively.

What might neo-Sabbatarian laws—laws that protect coordinated, rhythmic social time—look like? We have dedicated so few brain cells to the problem during the past half century that it's hard to envision the exact dimensions of a solution. Who knows what a team of crack labor-policy wonks might come up with? But if we do make the collective decision that this kind of time is worth protecting, two things should become apparent: one, that the market is unlikely to protect it for us, and two, that we have more tools at our disposal than simple legal proscriptions.

We could start by tackling overwork. We could adopt European Union vacation policies (a minimum of four weeks), shorter work-weeks (thirty-five hours, say), paid parental leave, and limits on over-time. We could emulate Germany and the Netherlands and give workers the right to reduce their hours and their pay, unless compa-nies can prove that this would constitute a hardship.

But while such reforms would help Americans balance work and family life, and might even generate jobs in this age of underemploy-ment, they don't address the problem of *coordinating* social time. It would be impossible, and probably undesirable, to forbid people to work at night or on weekends. But we could create a web of incen-tives and disincentives that might make it easier on those who do, and also remedy the harm done to society. We could tax off-hours labor and use the money to bolster the civic institutions weakened by the diminution of the pool of available volunteers. We could mandate higher pay or graduated bonuses for protracted or irregular schedules that reflect the hidden social and personal costs of staggered hours. We could strengthen a worker's right to refuse overtime or a job reassign-ment that entailed working non-standard hours.

Each of these measures might have negative and unforeseen con-sequences, and we should instruct our labor-policy wonks to model all possible outcomes. And we should concede that a full day of rest in the global era is probably a fantasy. But Henry Ward Beecher was right: The idea does have uplift. Who thinks in terms of preserving public culture anymore? Everybody talks about popular culture, but pop culture is a creature of segmented markets, not common ones. Sunday once gave Americans an experience that was national in scope, personal in character, and religiously neutral. As soon as reli-gion was disestablished, no one had to go to church—or anywhere else, for that matter.

As for the common day of rest falling on Sunday, Frankfurter, in *McGowan et al. v. Maryland,* pointed out that to share a day of rest, you had to pick one, and it might as well be the one that most people already observed. The secular Sunday was implicitly a national holiday. One day a week—it is worth remembering—the country honored life beyond duty and the imperatives of the marketplace. For twenty-four hours, we stayed home and ate huge family dinners, or went to church, or set off on afternoon drives. And we not only did these things with members of our inner circle; we did them with the knowledge that everyone else was doing them, too. That gave us permission not to work, too, along with the rest of the nation. We had fewer choices, but that lack of choice, in retrospect, was liberating, because our inexhaustible options trail behind them the realization that we're not doing everything we could be doing. We embraced laziness, goofiness, random reading, desultory conversation, neighbors and relatives both pleasant and unpleasant—the kinds of things that knit us together even as they made us more ourselves.

7.

THE CONVENTIONS of spiritual autobiography require me to conclude by telling you how I keep the Sabbath now, as opposed to when I began this book. The answer is, I have not changed all that much, and everything has changed for me. I keep the Sabbath, but only halfway—by strict Jewish standards, at least—which sometimes feels fine and sometimes feels shameful but has come to feel inevitable.

My husband and I work hard at the celebratory aspects of the Sabbath. We spend the week scouring farmers' markets for fresh fruits and vegetables, and on Friday mornings and afternoons we make an elaborate dinner, and sometimes, if we get home in time, take baths and dress up, and we invite friends over or we go to their homes, and we light the candles, and we bless the children, the wine, the challah, and the washing of our hands. As for the negative proscriptions—the "do nots"—we observe those largely by keeping our electronic devices off, including cell phones. These we use only if we *really, really* need to. We put our wallets away, with the same resolution about money, which is not to be handled on the Sabbath.

But we live in New York City, and amid the many temptations it's easy to confuse need with desire. We no longer drive to synagogue, but sometimes the children's whining about the thirteen-block walk forces us into a cab, which entails driving *and* handling money. The period after services poses a problem, and on those winter days when we have failed to wangle an invitation to someone's home for lunch or lack the energy to put on a spread ourselves, when the seconds tick slowly and the children grow restless, we go to a museum. In that case, we may not have to pay—we can usually go to the ones at which we can flash membership cards—but we're sure to take our wallets back out when it comes to buying food, drink, maybe even toys. I recently confronted the specter of Saturday-morning soccer practice, and was defeated by it. My son now plays soccer instead of going to synagogue, and my husband goes with him.

I feel guilty about not building better fences around the day, but apparently not guilty enough. Partly, it's because each step up in observance paralyzes me with indecision. Why follow this rule and not that one? Where to begin? But also, I think, it's because my religious commitments remain too abstract to overcome the inconvenience of making them. Probably the only way for me to trick myself into being *shomer Shabbat* would be to restrict myself to circles where such behavior is the norm, not subject to constant question.

Anyway, I still like the idea of the fully observed Sabbath more than I like observing it. I like the idea of being commanded, too, in the same ambivalent way, because I believe that I am. Being commanded strikes me as a succinct way of saying "being born into the world." Being commanded means that customs come upon us from the outside, like the language that we learn from our parents, and from the inside, like the still small voice of conscience. What others call God, I call ritual.

I like to think that I share this view with Kafka. At least that's how I read his famous parable of the leopards:

Leopards break into the temple and drink the sacrificial chalices dry; this occurs repeatedly, again and again: finally it can be reckoned on beforehand and becomes a part of the ceremony.

In one run-on sentence Kafka provides a history of ritual, a definition of God, and a theory of habit. *Ritual* tames the trauma caused by the leopards—the random violence of life—by incorporating them into a routine. *Religion* is the sum of such routines. *God* is what we make of the leopards. After all, the wine in the sacrificial chalices had been set aside for God. If leopards drink the wine again and again, and if that action has become central to a ritual script, then according to that script leopards play the part of God. And if they do that, why then, soon enough, we're bound to perceive them *as* God, or as gods. And very good gods they make, too: terrifying, beautiful, unpredictable, susceptible to domestication.

God, then, is the ungovernable reality commemorated by ritual. Ritual reflects the highly contingent anthropological, geographical, agricultural, and historical facts that conditioned our neural pathways and tribal behaviors and the forms and customs that became religion, and that even now determine through force of repetition the way things ought to be. Or maybe I've just naïvely inflated a random evolutionary outcome—the human predisposition to incarnate memory in custom, and those customs themselves—into an overblown fantasy called God. God, then, is my parents, and my parents' parents, and all those who came before. God is the ancestors, which is probably how our ancestors saw the matter.

Not long ago, my six-year-old son, Moses, a boy with many reservations about his Jewish-day-school education, informed me, with genuine sorrow, that he didn't believe in God. "Sometimes," he said, "I think God is a story someone made up a long time ago and told to his children, and his children told it to his children, and so on, until we all got into the habit of thinking it was true." Though sometimes, he added, he thinks that he's wrong, and that God will punish him harshly for daring to think such things.

I realized with chagrin that I am one of Moses' children, in all the senses of that phrase. I tell the story of God to my children so that they will tell it to their children. I keep the Sabbath more or less the way my parents kept it, and chances are that my children will keep it more or less the same way. Actually, I suspect that my Moses will not keep it at all, but that, too, is a part of his heritage, a way for him to stay loyal to me. Will the ancestors take revenge on him, as he fears they will? Probably. They did on me. I grapple with them every Saturday.

Freud also thought ritual—which he equated with obsessive-compulsiveness and neurosis—was the revenge of the dead. In *Totem and Taboo,* he gave his Oedipal history of religion: It came into being when a group of brothers killed their father, who had denied them access to women. Instantly, they felt remorse. Their guilt required expiation, so they invented ritual as a form of self-punishment. They also ate the father, an event that becomes the basis for religious festivals, and everything else besides. The totem meal, Freud wrote, was "a repetition and a commemoration of this memorable and criminal deed," as well as "the beginning of so many things—of social organization, of moral restrictions and of religion."

The autobiographical moment for which this fantasy is said to have been a screen can be found in *The Interpretation of Dreams.* Here Freud tells a tale that is usually characterized as one of his earliest encounters with anti-Semitism and, therefore, a primal scene that explains his defensively dismissive attitude toward religion. Curiously, it's also a tale of the Sabbath. When Freud was ten or twelve years old, he went on a walk with his father, Jakob Freud—perhaps a Sabbath walk, since Jakob was known to take them—during which Jakob told a story that was meant to explain to Sigmund that life had improved a great deal for Jews over the course of Jakob's lifetime. The events described in Jakob's story, in any case, definitely take place on a Sabbath walk:

"When I was a young man," said Jakob Freud, "I went for a walk one Saturday in the streets of your birthplace; I was well dressed, and had a new fur cap on my head. A Christian came up to me and with a single blow knocked off my cap into the mud and shouted: 'Jew! get off the pavement!' "

"And what did you do?" asked young Sigmund.

"I went into the roadway and picked up my cap," Jakob quietly replied.

The young Freud was dismayed: "This struck me as unheroic conduct on the part of the big, strong man who was holding the little boy by the hand." Whenever he thought about the incident, he substituted for the disturbing image of his submissive father another that he liked better: a scene in which the Carthaginian general Hannibal's father "made his boy swear before the household altar to take vengeance on the Romans."

Some background is required to understand all this. Jakob Freud was raised in a Hasidic family and well trained in Jewish literature and ritual; indeed, there is evidence that he homeschooled Sigmund until he was seven and taught him Hebrew, Torah, and Talmud, even though Freud sometimes denied having had enough Jewish education to distinguish Yiddish from Hebrew. Given Jakob's upbringing, it seems distinctly possible that the hat that was knocked off his head was a *shtreimel,* a round, flat ring of fur worn by Hasidic men on the Sabbath and on Jewish holidays. The *shtreimel,* if that's what Jakob Freud was wearing, was a flagrant display of ritual headgear; and if that is not what he was wearing, Jakob was still obviously dressed up for the Sabbath, a fact that would not have escaped his son.

This story, then, gives us another way to imagine the relationship between ritual and trauma, especially as Freud saw it. Ritual is not only an expiation for, or a defense against, trauma, as per *Totem and Taboo.* Ritual itself traumatizes. The singular Jewishness of Jakob Freud's Sabbath hat singled him out for violence. On six days he passed as a regular German (the incident took place in Freiburg, a town in what is now the Czech Republic, which is where the Freud family lived before they moved to Vienna); on the seventh day he was a Jew, and assaulted as such. What the story comes to teach us is that if ritual is born of trauma the aversion to ritual is also born of trauma—the trauma of ritual. Keeping the Sabbath as our forefathers did straitjackets us in an identity that we did not choose and for which we may not want to take the consequences. It goes against our yearning for a world of infinite possibility. It exposes us to violence, ridicule, prejudice, ostracism.

On the other hand, we are often as irrationally opposed to ritual as ritual is irrational in its demands upon us. Freud's marriage to his much-beloved Martha, who had been raised in a deeply observant Jewish home, nearly failed to take place because he refused to participate in a Jewish ceremony. Shortly thereafter, he forbade Martha to light the Sabbath candles, a bit of marital high-handedness that she remained bitter about throughout their otherwise apparently happy marriage. (She began lighting candles again after he died.)

Rituals are not just idealized visions of how things can be. They are also artifacts of history. Why choose Sunday as the American day of rest? Because that is what it has always been, and tradition has its virtues. Or maybe it doesn't. Maybe what the choice of Sunday commemorates is the rage and insecurity at the heart of Christianity about Jews and their Sabbath, feelings that had homicidal and even genocidal consequences. Maybe we ought not to honor so ignoble a history. Or maybe it is more honest to let Sunday continue to remind us of its problematic origins. The philosopher Jürgen Habermas once argued that one of the advantages of secular societies is that they substitute rational discourse or speech for the manipulatively symbolic communications of ritual. If you can discuss the way things should be, rather than simply enact your vision of them or let them impose their history on you, you have a hope of arriving at a reasoned, reflective consensus about the good life. Should we rest on Sunday or Saturday, or any day in seven? Let us hold a conference on the subject.

The problem with Habermas's Platonic reasonableness is that it would banish the poets, along with their poetry. The Sabbath may have defensible social value, in that it offers excellent ideas about time and society, but it also bears testimony to that which can't be defended, only re-experienced: men and women mute with the disjunctions of exile and the awkwardness of living in a time that does not feel like theirs and mournful with the wish to find a home, if not in space, then in time. And because the Sabbath, Sunday as well as Saturday, is a day those men and women kept, and not a conversation they had, the men and women who came after them remembered it. And when they, too, felt discomfited by their world, they were able to do something about that feeling and assuage their pain a bit. Or maybe they didn't do what they had been taught to do, because it no longer gave them comfort, but not doing while feeling uncomfortable about it is also a way of remembering.

So why remember the Sabbath? Because the Sabbath comes to us out of the past—out of the bodies of our mothers and fathers, out of the churches on our streets, out of our own dreams—to train us to pay attention to it. And why do we need to be trained? Consider the mystery surrounding God's first Sabbath. Why *did* God stop, anyway? In the eighteenth century, Rabbi Elijah of Vilna (the Vilna Gaon) ventured this explanation: God stopped to show us that what we create becomes meaningful only once we stop creating it and start remembering why it was worth creating in the first place. Or—if this is the thought to which our critical impulses lead us—why it *wasn't* worth creating, why it isn't up to snuff and should be created anew. After all, God, contemplating his first Creation, decided to destroy it in a flood. We could let the world wind us up and set us to working, like dolls that go until they fall over because they have no way of stopping. But that would make us less than human. We have to remember to stop because we have to stop to remember.

NOTES

INTRODUCTION THE VIEW FROM AFAR

xiv "is perfectly *sui generis* and irreducible": Rudolf Otto, *The Idea of the Holy,* translated by John W. Harvey (New York, London: Oxford University Press, 1923), p. 7.

xv The Law, the legal theorist: Robert Cover, "Nomos and Narrative," *Harvard Law Review* 97, no. 1 (November 1983): 4–69.

xv "Holy days, rituals, liturgies": Yosef Hayim Yerushalmi, *Zakhor: Jewish History and Jewish Memory* (Seattle: University of Washington Press for Jewish Publication Society of America, 1982), pp. 42–43.

xvi "Because of the river Sambatyon": Sanhedrin 65b; Genesis Rabbah 11:5.

xvii "for they have no manservants": Elkan Nathan Adler, ed., *Jewish Travellers* (London: George Routledge & Sons, 1930), p. 13.

xviii "Sunday comes, and brings": Charles Dickens, *Sunday, Under Three Heads* (London: J. W. Jarvis, 1836), p. 29.

xviii "In the Universe of Shabbat": Dov Peretz Elkins, ed., *A Shabbat Reader: Universe of Cosmic Joy* (New York: UAHC Press, 1998), p. xv.

xviii "the most brilliant creation": Quoted in Yedidia D. Stern, "From a Shabbat of Work to a Shabbat of Rest," Israeli Democracy Institute website, February 26, 2007, http://www.idi.org.il/sites/english/

ResearchAndPrograms/ReligionandState/Pages/ReligionandState
Article2FromaShabbat.aspx.

xxi "religious behaviorism": Abraham Joshua Heschel, *Moral Grandeur
and Spiritual Audacity: Essays* (New York: Farrar, Straus & Giroux, 1996),
pp. 104–5.

xxii "a knight of faith": Søren Kierkegaard, *Fear and Trembling: Dialectical
Lyric by Johannes de Silentio,* translated by Alastair Hannay (New York:
Penguin, 1985), pp. 68 ff.

xxiii "necessarily associated with": Max Kadushin, *The Rabbinic Mind* (Jewish Theological Seminary of America, 1952), p. 169.

xxv "the ordinary man": Franz Kafka, *Letters to Friends, Family and Editors,*
translated by Richard and Clara Winston (New York: Schocken Books,
1977), p. 285.

xxv "would be ready to fulfill": Franz Kafka, *Parables and Paradoxes,* in German and English, edited by Nahum H. Glatzer (New York: Schocken
Books, 1961 [1935]), pp. 42–43.

xxvi "The Sabbath was made": Mark 2:27.

xxvii "When the time for Jumu'ah": Abdullah Yusuf Ali, *The Meaning of the
Holy Qur'an* (Brentwood, Md.: Amana Publications, 1999), p. 1469,
footnote 5462.

xxvii "There are one hundred and fifty-seven": Haim Nachman Bialik, *Halacha and Agada* (London: Zionist Federation of Great Britain and Ireland, 1944), p. 12, cited in Yosef Yitzhak Lifshitz, "Secrets of the
Sabbath," *Azure,* no. 10 (Winter 2001): 86.

xxx "Only from the inside": Alice Munro, *The View from Castle Rock: Stories*
(New York: Random House, 2007), p. 17.

PART ONE TIME SICKNESS

4 "from sunset": Babylonian Talmud, *Shabbat* 34b.

4 The story is told: *Pirkei Avot,* 5:8.

4 Is it still twilight?: Babylonian Talmud, *Shabbat* 34b.

8 The Talmud asks: Babylonian Talmud, *Shabbat* 69b.

10 "mostly *headaches* or *stomach disturbances*": Sándor Ferenczi, *Further Contributions to the Theory and Technique of Psychoanalysis,* translated by Jane
Isabel Suttie and others (New York: Boni & Liveright, 1927), pp.
174–77.

11 "So long as man marked": Daniel Boorstin, *The Discoverers: A History of
Man's Search to Know His World and Himself* (New York: Random
House, 1983), p. 12.

12 "Sunday is the holiday": Ferenczi, *Further Contributions,* p. 175.

13   "psychological man": Philip Rieff, *The Triumph of the Therapeutic* (New York: Harper & Row, 1966).

15   "My father, who": Quoted in Frederick C. Beiser and Mary Gluck, *Georg Lukács and His Generation, 1900–1918* (Cambridge: Harvard University Press, 1991), p. 70.

16   the cultural historian: Stephen Kern, *The Culture of Time and Space: 1880–1918* (Cambridge: Harvard University Press, 1983), pp. 1–65.

17   To maximize the time spent: Arlie Russell Hochschild, *The Time Bind: When Work Becomes Home and Home Becomes Work* (New York: Metropolitan Books, 1997).

18   She based this on: Juliet Schor, *The Overworked American: The Unexpected Decline of Leisure* (New York: Basic Books, 1991).

18   You acknowledge that: John P. Robinson and Geoffrey Godbey, *Time for Life: The Surprising Ways Americans Use Their Time* (University Park: Pennsylvania State University Press, 1997).

18   "in the evening, at night": Harriet B. Presser, *Working in a 24/7 Economy: Challenges for American Families* (New York: Russell Sage Foundation, 2003), p. 1.

20   "The clock, not the steam-engine": Lewis Mumford, *Technics and Civilization* (New York: Harcourt, Brace, 1934), p. 14.

20   According to the British: E. P. Thompson, "Time, Work-Discipline, and Industrial Capitalism," *Past & Present,* no. 38 (December 1967): 56–97.

20   "The infraction of its rules": Max Weber, *The Protestant Ethic and the Spirit of Capitalism,* translated by Talcott Parsons (Mineola, N.Y.: Dover, 2003), p. 51.

21   "We had always": Staffan Burenstam Linder, *The Harried Leisure Class* (New York: Columbia University Press, 1970), pp. 1 ff.

22   Scheuch called this: Quoted in Thomas Goodale and Geoffrey Godbey, *The Evolution of Leisure: Historical and Philosophical Perspectives* (State College, Penn.: Venture Publishing, 1988), p. 127.

22   Lacking the leisure: Linder, *The Harried Leisure Class,* p. 71.

23   "Despite school times": Thompson, "Time, Work-Discipline, and Industrial Capitalism," p. 79.

24   In 1973: John M. Darley and C. Daniel Batson, "From Jerusalem to Jericho: A Study of Situational and Dispositional Variables in Helping Behavior," *Journal of Personality and Social Psychology* 27 (1973): 100–108.

27   "Call the Sabbath a delight": Isaiah 58:16.

27   "When the Holy Temple": Babylonian Talmud, *Pesachim* 109b.

27   "This cup is the new": Luke 22:20.

27   Everyone swigs wine in the Bible: Elliott Horowitz, "Sabbath Delights:
      Towards a Social History," in *Sabbath: Idea, History, Reality,* edited by
      Gerald J. Blidstein (Beer Sheva, Israel: Ben Gurion University of the
      Negev Press, 2004), pp. 131–58.

28   "Work makes for prosperous days": Charles Baudelaire, "Du Vin et du
      Haschisch," in *Les Paradis Artificiels,* vol. 1 (Paris: Bibliothèque de la
      Pléiade, Gallimard, 1975), p. 380.

28   "Every person": Abraham H. Lewis, *A Critical History of Sunday Legis-
      lation from 321 to 1888 A.D.* (New York: D. Appleton, 1888), p. 22, cited
      in David N. Laband and Deborah Hendry Heinbuch, *Blue Laws: The
      History, Economics, and Politics of Sunday-Closing Laws, 1987* (Lexington,
      Mass.: Lexington Books, 1987), pp. 18–19.

29   "communitas": Victor Turner, *The Ritual Process: Structure and Anti-
      Structure* (Chicago: Aldine, 1969), pp. 94 ff.

30   "Community is the being": Martin Buber, *The Martin Buber Reader: Es-
      sential Writings* (New York: Palgrave Macmillan, 2002), p. 201.

PART TWO GROUP DYNAMICS

32   "The emotion seems too raw": David Rosenberg, ed., *Congregation:
      Contemporary Writers Read the Hebrew Bible* (New York: Harcourt Brace
      Jovanovich, 1987), p. 384.

32   On the contrary: Amy Docker Marcus, *The View from Nebo: How Ar-
      chaeology Is Rewriting the Bible and Reshaping the Middle East* (Boston:
      Back Bay Press, 2001), p. 157.

32   "The tongue of the suckling": Lamentations 4:4–5.

32   "Those who feasted on dainties": Lamentations 2:20.

32   "But the Babylonian troups": 2 Kings 25:7.

33   "slew all the nobles": Jeremiah 39:6.

33   "poorest in the land": 2 Kings 25:11.

33   "The foe has laid hands": Lamentations 1:10.

33   "All who admired her": Lamentations 1:8–9.

33   "He has broken my teeth": Lamentations 3:16.

35   "is both ingenious": Roland de Vaux, *Ancient Israel* (New York:
      McGraw-Hill, 1965), p. 479.

35   "when the gods' heart": Ibid., p. 476.

36   "For a people in ancient times": Yosef Hayim Yerushalmi, *Zakhor: Jew-
      ish History and Jewish Memory* (Seattle: University of Washington Press
      for Jewish Publication Society of America, 1982), p. 13.

36   "are grounded in": Émile Durkheim, *The Elementary Forms of Religious
      Life,* translated by Karen E. Fields (New York: Free Press, 1995), p. 2.

36   "Although religious thought": Ibid., p. 385.

38   "freedom of time regime": Todd D. Rakoff, *A Time for Every Purpose: Law and the Balance of Life* (Cambridge: Harvard University Press, 2002), pp. 157 ff.

39   "If, for example": Ibid., p. 161.

41   "because ye sanctified": Deuteronomy 32:51.

41   "Would to God": Exodus 16:2–3.

41   "walk in my law": Exodus 16:4.

42   "against Moses": Exodus 15:24.

42   "for them a statute": Exodus 15:25.

42   "wafers made with honey": Exodus 16:31.

42   "What is it but heavenly": Ilana Pardes, *The Biography of Ancient Israel* (Berkeley: University of California Press, 2000), p. 51.

43   "And it came to pass": Exodus 16:27–30.

43   "The man shall be": Numbers 15:35.

44   "cut off from among": Exodus 31:14.

45   "because the next day": *The Jeruslaem Post,* December 13, 2002.

46   "affords men leisure to meet": Saadia Gaon, *The Book of Beliefs and Opinions,* translated by Samuel Rosenblatt (New Haven, Conn.: Yale University Press, 1948), p. 143.

47   "a day peculiarly American": Henry Ward Beecher, "Libraries and Public Reading Rooms: Should They Be Opened on Sunday?" (Cambridge, Mass.: J. Ford, 1872).

47   "moral earnestness": Elwood Worcester, "Shall We Keep Sunday or Lose It?" 1906.

48   "a cultural asset": *McGowan et al. v. Maryland,* 366 U.S. 420 (1961).

48   "He is my shepherd": Isaiah 44:28.

48   It should be noted: Joseph Blenkinsopp, "Temple and Society in Achaemenid Judah," in *Second Temple Studies, Persian Period,* vol. 1, edited by Philip R. Davies, *Journal for the Study of the Old Testament,* Supplement Series 117 (Sheffield, England: Sheffield Academic Press, 1991), p. 47.

49   "In those days": Nehemiah 13:15–22.

50   "It was also": C. C. McCown, "City," in *The Interpreter's Dictionary of the Bible,* vol. 1, edited by George Arthur Buttrick (Nashville, Tenn.: Abingdon, 1962), p. 634.

50   "Thus cleansed": Nehemiah 13:30.

53   "like prodigal sons": Jonathan Sarna, *American Judaism* (New Haven, Conn.: Yale University Press, 2004), pp. 266–68.

54   Influential friends: Robert Trotter, "Muzafer Sherif: A Life of Conflict and Goals," *Psychology Today,* September 1985, pp. 55–59.

54   Anyone who has lived: Muzafer Sherif and Carolyn W. Sherif, *An Outline of Social Psychology* (New York: Harper & Brothers, 1956), pp. 301 ff.

55   The campers "perceived": Amy Sales and Leonard Saxe, *How Goodly Are Thy Tents* (Lebanon, N.H.: University Press of New England, 2004), p. 3.

55   from the beginning: Abigail Van Slyck, *A Manufactured Wilderness: Summer Camps and the Shaping of American Youth, 1890–1960* (Minneapolis: University of Minnesota Press, 2006).

PART THREE THE SCANDAL OF THE HOLY

60   "The word *Sabbath*": Thomas Shepard, *The Works of Thomas Shepard,* vol. 3, *Theses Sabbaticae* (Ligonier, Penn.: Soli Deo Gloria Publications, 1992), p. 254.

61   "What is the origin": Émile Durkheim, *The Elementary Forms of Religious Life,* translated by Karen E. Fields (New York: Free Press, 1995), pp. 9–10.

61   "The sacred thing is": Ibid., p. 56.

62   "There is no religion": Ibid., p. 347.

62   "All over the world": Edmund R. Leach, "Two Essays Concerning the Symbolic Representation of Time," in *Rethinking Anthropology* (Oxford: Berg Publishers, 1966), pp. 132 ff.

64   "Divine election is an exacting": Robert Alter, *The World of Biblical Literature* (New York: Basic Books, 1992), p. 105.

64   "Holiness means keeping": Mary Douglas, *Purity and Danger* (New York: Routledge, 1966), p. 67.

64   "a principle of separation": David Damrosch, "Leviticus," in *The Literary Guide to the Bible,* edited by Robert Alter and Frank Kermode (Cambridge: Harvard University Press, 1987), p. 74.

67   "The Tabernacle": Numbers Rabbah 12:13.

69   "It is like a man": Bereshit Rabbah 10:9.

70   "This may be compared": Ibid.

71   "We may eat": Genesis 3:2 ff.

71   "the question is rhetorical": *Genesis,* translated by E. A. Speiser (New York: Doubleday, 1962), p. 24.

71   "God knew": *The Metsudah Chumash/Rashi,* vol. 1, translated by Rabbi Avrohom Davis ("Bereishis") (Israel Book Shop, 2002), p. 34.

72   "They had enjoyed": Louis Ginzberg, *The Legends of the Jews* (Baltimore: Johns Hopkins University Press, 1998), p. 82.

73   "What was there": Samson Raphael Hirsch, *Horeb: A Philosophy of Jew-*

ish Laws and Observances, translated by Dayan Dr. I. Grunfeld (New York: Soncino Press, 1994), pp. 62 ff.

75   "correspond to the basic": All quotes from Arendt are from Hannah Arendt, *The Human Condition* (Chicago: University of Chicago Press, 1998), pp. 7 ff.

77   In 167 B.C.E.: My source for this narrative and the quotes within it is the Anchor Bible's *I Maccabees* and *II Maccabees,* as well as the introductions and notes by the editor, Jonathan Goldstein (New York: Doubleday, 1976).

80   "will appear to such": Josephus, *Against Apion,* in *The New Complete Works of Josephus,* vol. 1, translated by William Whiston (Grand Rapids, Mich.: Kregel, 1999), 949, 209–12.

81   "speak great words": Daniel 7:25.

81   "many of them that sleep": Daniel 12:2–3.

82   "They had learned": Yosef Hayim Yerushalmi, *Zakhor: Jewish History and Jewish Memory* (Seattle: University of Washington Press for Jewish Publication Society of America, 1982), p. 21.

PART FOUR   THE FLIGHT FROM TIME

92   "Let us alone": All quotes in this scene from Mark 1.

93   "Mark's Jesus": Paula Fredriksen, *Jesus of Nazareth: King of the Jews* (New York: Alfred A. Knopf, 1999), p. 31.

93   "Apocalypse hovers": Harold Bloom, *Jesus and Yahweh* (New York: Riverhead Books, 2005), pp. 60 ff.

93   "cosmic apocalyptic eschatological": *Mark 1–8: A New Translation with Introduction and Commentary by Joel Marcus* (New York: Doubleday, 2000), p. 72. (Marcus attributes the phrase to a Dutch Bible scholar named M. C. de Boer.)

94   "The time is short": 1 Corinthians 7:29.

96   "space of flows": Manuel Castells, *The Rise of the Network Society* (London: Blackwell, 2000), p. 445.

97   "the man of science": Henry Adams, *The Education of Henry Adams: An Autobiography* (Boston: Houghton Mifflin, 1918), pp. 486–87.

98   "a new series of time": Frank Kermode, *The Sense of an Ending: Studies in the Theory of Fiction* (New York: Oxford University Press, 2000), p. 188.

98   "the fulness of the time": Galatians 4:4.

98   "the pivotal concept": Søren Kierkegaard, *The Concept of Anxiety: A Simple Psychologically Orienting Deliberation on the Dogmatic Issue of Hereditary Sin,* edited and translated by Reidar Thomte, in collabora-

tion with Albert B. Anderson (Princeton, N.J.: Princeton University Press, 1980), p. 90.

98   "Have you ever had a gallop": C. S. Lewis, *The Lion, the Witch and the Wardrobe* (New York: HarperCollins, 1978), pp. 180–81.

101   In one such study: Hogne Øian, "Time Out and Drop Out: On the Relation Between Linear Time and Individualism," *Time and Society* 13, no. 2/3 (2004): 173–94.

107   "What we now think": Fredriksen, *Jesus of Nazareth,* p. 130.

107   "You make yourself a laughing-stock": Origen, *Contra Celsum* 7.36, quoted in Robert Wilken, *John Chrysostom and the Jews: Rhetoric and Reality in the Late 4th Century* (Berkeley: University of California Press, 1983), p. 139.

107   " 'Who is my mother?' ": Matthew 12:48–50.

109   "There is neither Jew": Galatians 3:28.

109   "days, and months": Galatians 4:10.

109   "After that ye have known": Galatians 4:9.

109   "Sabbatizing": Samuele Bacchiocchi, *From Sabbath to Sunday: A Historical Investigation of the Rise of Sunday Observance in Early Christianity* (Rome: Pontifical Gregorian University Press, 1977), p. 214.

109   "because of your sins": Justin Martyr, *Dialogue with Trypho,* translated by Thomas B. Falls (New York: Christian Heritage, 1948), p. 175.

110   "was that you": Ibid., p. 188.

110   "Thou shalt eat neither swine": Barnabas, *The Epistle of Barnabas,* in *The Didache, The Epistle of Barnabas, The Epistles and The Martyrdom of St. Polycarp, The Fragments of Papias, The Epistle to Diognetus,* translated by James A. Kleist (Westminster, Md.: Newman Press, 1961), pp. 50–51.

111   "And on the day": Justin Martyr, "The First Apology of Justin Martyr," in *Early Christian Fathers,* edited by Cyril Richardson (Philadelphia: Westminster Press, 1953), pp. 242 ff.

112   One student of Sunday: Willy Rordorf, *Sunday: The History of the Day of Rest and Worship in the Earliest Centuries of the Christian Church,* translated by A.A.K. Graham (Philadelphia: Westminster Press, 1968), pp. 157–59.

112   Nothing could be less: Bacchiocchi, *From Sabbath to Sunday,* p. 187.

113   Worried that his prisoners: Pliny, *The Letters of the Younger Pliny,* translated by Betty Radice (New York: Penguin, 1969), p. 294.

114   In a book titled: Both the narrative and the quotes that follow are taken from Robert Wilken, *John Chrysostom and the Jews: Rhetoric and Reality in the Late 4th Century* (Berkeley: University of California Press, 1983).

PART FIVE PEOPLE OF THE BOOK

120 "Printing," he declared: Martin Luther, M. Luthers *Werke: Kritische Gesamtausgabe* (Weimar: H. Böhlau, 1883–), quoted and translated by Jean-François Gilmont in *The Reformation and the Book,* edited by Jean-François Gilmont and translated by Karin Maag (Brookfield, Vt.: Ashgate, 1998), p. 1.

120 "a truly mass readership": Lucien Febvre and Henri-Jean Martin, *The Coming of the Book: The Impact of Printing, 1450–1800,* translated by David Gerard (London: Verso, 1997), p. 295.

120 One study of a mining: Gilmont, *The Reformation and the Book,* p. 86.

121 And then there were the wives: P. Imbart de la Tour, *Les Origines de la Reforme,* vol. 4 (Paris: Librairie Hachette, 1909–1935), quoted ibid., pp. 225, 264.

122 "there were biblical": Fania Oz-Salzberger, "The Jewish Roots of Western Freedom," *Azure,* no. 13 (2002): 88–132.

123 "therefore could not be coterminous": Daniel Liechty, *Andreas Fischer and the Sabbatarian Anabaptists* (Scottsdale, Penn., & Kitchener, Ohio: Herald Press, 1988), p. 108.

124 The key fact about the Radical Reformation: Daniel Liechty, *Sabbatarianism in the Sixteenth Century* (Berrien Springs, Mich.: Andrews University Press, 1993), p. 5.

125 "unlearned," "foolish," "apes," and "Judaizers": Martin Luther, *M. Luthers Werke,* vol. 50, pp. 312–37.

125 "went thrice as far as the Jews": John Calvin, *Institutes of the Christian Religion,* translated by Henry Beveridge (Grand Rapids, Mich.: William B. Eerdmans, 1957), pp. 28–34.

126 "Christ did not come": Liechty, *Andreas Fischer and the Sabbatarian Anabaptists,* p. 103.

126 the influence of Christian Hebraism: Its history and ideas are recounted in Jerome Friedman, *The Most Ancient Testimony: Sixteenth-Century Christian-Hebraica in the Age of Renaissance Nostalgia* (Athens: Ohio University Press, 1983).

127 "Not only Mohammedans and Hebrews": Ibid., p. 61.

128 the Transylvanian *Szombatosok:* I base my account of the *Szombatosok* on the following sources: W. Bacher, "The Sabbatarians in Hungary," *Jewish Quarterly Review* 2, no. 4 (July 1890): 465–93; Moshe Carmelly-Weinberger, "A Northern Transylvanian Tale: Days When Proselytes Shared Martyrdom of Jews," *Martyrdom and Resistance* 16, no. 3 (Jan.-Feb. 1990); *Antitrinitarianism in the Second Half of the 16th Century,* edited by Róbert Dán and Antal Pirnát (Budapest: Akadémiai Kiadó;

Leiden: E. J. Brill, 1982); Judit Gellérd, "Spiritual Jews of Szekler Jerusalem: A Four-Centuries History of Transylvanian Szekler Sabbatarianism," unpublished paper, 2000; Liechty, *Sabbatarianism in the Sixteenth Century;* Kenneth Strand, *The Sabbath in Scripture and History* (Washington, D.C.: Review and Herald Publishing Association, 1982); Earl Morse Wilbur, *A History of Unitarianism in Transylvania, England, and America* (Boston: Beacon Press, 1945).

129 "the greatest debate in the entire history of Unitarianism": Wilbur, *A History of Unitarianism in Transylvania, England, and America,* p. 36.

130 "This man": W. Bacher, "The Sabbatarians in Hungary," *Jewish Quarterly Review* 2, no. 4 (July 1890), p. 472.

130 "abstain[ed] from blood and pork": Judit Gellérd, "Spiritual Jews of Szekler Jerusalem: A Four-Centuries History of Transylvanian Szekler Sabbatarianism," unpublished paper, 2000.

132 "The thirty-eight Sabbatarian": Bacher, "The Sabbatarians in Hungary," p. 484.

133 After four hundred years: Gellérd, "Spiritual Jews of Szekler Jerusalem."

134 "Am not I": All of the following can be found in the first two chapters of 1 Samuel.

135 "You do not know": Babylonian Talmud, *Berachot* 31b.

135 "How many important laws": Babylonian Talmud, *Berachot* 31a.

138 "dead drunke": The following is taken from Thomas Shepard, *God's Plot: The Paradoxes of Puritan Piety. Being the Autobiography and Journal of Thomas Shepard,* edited by Michael McGiffert (Amherst: University of Massachusetts Press, 1972).

141 "a bit of English originality": M. M. Knappen, *Tudor Puritanism* (Chicago: University of Chicago Press, 1969), p. 142.

141 "the industrious sort of people": Christopher Hill, *Society and Puritanism in Pre-Revolutionary England* (Palgrave Macmillan, 1997), p. 107.

141 "the mother and breeder": Christopher Hill, *Society and Puritanism in Pre-Revolutionary England* (New York: Palgrave Macmillan, 1997), pp. 137 ff.

142 "How were men to be reorganized": Michael Walzer, *The Revolution of the Saints: A Study in the Origins of Radical Politics* (Cambridge: Harvard University Press, 1965), pp. 202 ff.

142 "Biblical primitivism": Theodore Dwight Bozeman, *To Live Ancient Lives: The Primitivist Dimension in Puritanism* (Chapel Hill: University of North Carolina Press, 1988).

143 the Puritan Sabbath was the product: I base my discussion of Puritan Sabbatarian theology on John H. Primus, *Holy Time: Moderate Puritanism and the Sabbath* (Macon, Ga.: Mercer University Press, 1989).

144 "his primitive and perfect estate": Thomas Shepard, *The Works of Thomas Shepard,* vol. 3, *Theses Sabbaticae* (Ligonier, Penn.: Soli Deo Gloria Publications, 1992), p. 41.

144 "to bring ourselves back into that estate": Nicholas Bownde, *The Doctrine of the Sabbath* (London: Printed by the Widdow Orwin, for Iohn Porter, and Thomas Man, 1595), p. 19.

145 "would say, they had seen": All the quotes in this paragraph from Samuel Clarke, *General Martyrologie* (Glasgow: J. Galbraith, 1770), quoted in William Haller, *The Rise of Puritanism* (New York: Harper & Brothers, 1957), p. 62.

145 "Psalm-singing replaced ballads": David D. Hall, *Worlds of Wonder, Days of Judgment: Popular Religious Belief in Early New England* (Cambridge: Harvard University Press, 1989), pp. 10 ff.

145 "state and royal majesty": Ibid.

146 "buying, selling, soweing": Ibid., pp. 257–58.

146 "Sweet to the Pilgrims": Alice Morse Earle, *The Sabbath in Puritan New England* (New York: Charles Scribner's Sons, 1891), pp. 257–58.

146 On Saturday night: Ibid., pp. 19–116.

147 The first Puritan colony: Most of the following can be found in Winston U. Solberg, *Redeem the Time: The Puritan Sabbath in Early America* (Cambridge: Harvard University Press, 1977), pp. 167–96.

149 "Children, servants, strangers": Shepard, *Theses Sabbaticae,* p. 263.

149 "And if superiors in families": Ibid.

150 "to be forever banished": Shepard, *Theses Sabbaticae,* p. 261.

150 "It would be no exaggeration": Gershom Scholem, *On the Kabbalah and Its Symbolism* (New York: Schocken Books, 1996), p. 139.

151 Consider the Sabbath: Elliot K. Ginsburg, *The Sabbath in the Classical Kabbalah* (Albany: State University of New York Press, 1989), pp. 217 ff.

152 "the other, holy spirit": Ibid., p. 131.

152 "Three things were said": Moe'ed Katan, 18a.

152 Isaac Luria, the great Kabbalist: Lawrence Fine, *Physician of the Soul, Healer of the Cosmos: Isaac Luria and His Kabbalistic Fellowship* (Palo Alto, Calif.: Stanford University Press, 2003), pp. 161–62.

153 And they had sex: Ibid., pp. 248–58.

153 "If the whole universe": Gershom Scholem, *Major Trends in Jewish Mysticism* (New York: Schocken Books, 1946), pp. 29–30.

155 Saint Augustine, as he lay weeping on the ground: Saint Augustine, *The Confessions,* translated by Maria Boulding (New York: Vintage, 1998), p. 168.

PART SIX SCENES OF INSTRUCTION

162 "Moses received": *Pirkei Avot,* 1:1.

162 "Rabbi Akiva said": Babylonian Talmud, *Berachot* 62a.

162 "Rabbi Kahana once went": Ibid.

164 They kept their eyes fixed: Laura Ingalls Wilder, *Little House in the Big Woods* (New York: HarperCollins, 2004), pp. 88–90.

164 "maddening church bells": Charles Dickens, *Little Dorrit* (London: J. M. Dent, 1899), pp. 39–43.

165 "never was late at Sabbath school": Mark Twain, *The Complete Short Stories of Mark Twain* (New York: Doubleday, 1985), pp. 67–70.

165 English and American Sabbath sentiment: The discussion of nineteenth-century Sabbatarianism is drawn from Alexis McCrossen, *Holy Day, Holiday: The American Sunday* (Ithaca, N.Y.: Cornell University Press, 2002); and John Wigley, *The Rise and Fall of the Victorian Sunday* (Manchester, England: Manchester University Press, 1980).

166 "my mother confined me": James Boswell, *The Life of Samuel Johnson, LL. D.* (London: G. Cowie, 1824), p. 56.

166 "Gaming-Tables, Night-Houses, Bawdy Houses": Thomas Legg, "Low-Life, or One Half of the World Knows Not How the Other Half Lives. Being a critical account of what is transacted by people of almost all religions, nations, circumstances, and sizes of understanding, between Saturday-night and Monday-morning" (London: Printed for the author, 1755?).

167 "The protest was unprecedented": Richard R. John, "Taking Sabbatarianism Seriously: The Postal System, the Sabbath, and the Transformation of American Political Culture," *Journal of the Early Republic* 1, no. 4 (Winter 1990): 517–67.

170 "a significant impact": Thomas Laqueur, *Religion and Respectability: Sunday Schools and Working Class Culture, 1780–1850* (New Haven, Conn.: Yale University Press, 1976), p. 123.

170 "religious terrorism": W.E.H. Lecky, *History of England in the Eighteenth Century,* vol. 2 (1891), p. 585.

170 "the neglect of moral discipline": E. P. Thompson, *The Making of the English Working Class* (New York: Vintage, 1966), p. 361.

170 "I . . . said that I had": Anne Stott, *Hannah More: The First Victorian* (Oxford: Oxford University Press, 2003), pp. 108 ff.

171 "I got a washing": Charles Shaw, *When I Was a Child,* by an Old Potter (London: Methuen, 1903), pp. 7–8.

171 "two different worlds": Ibid., p. 35.

172 "Let our Sunday schools": Laqueur, *Religion and Respectability,* pp. 154 ff.

173 "Here and there": Charles Dickens, *Sunday, Under Three Heads* (London: J. W. Jarvis & Son, 1836), pp. 3–4.

174 "Some keep the Sabbath": Emily Dickinson, *Poems: Including Variant Readings Critically Compared with All Known Manuscripts*, edited by Thomas Herbert Johnson (Cambridge: Belknap Press of Harvard University Press, 1955), p. 254.

175 "Childhood is unknown": Jean-Jacques Rousseau, *Emile, or On Education*, translated by Allan Bloom (New York: Basic Books, 1979), p. 33.

175 In the fifth of his *Reveries:* Jean-Jacques Rousseau, *Les confessions de J. J. Rousseau, suives Des reveries du promeneur solitaire*, vol. 2 (Geneva: N.p., 1783), pp. 285–303.

176 "slackening my thoughts by choice": All quotes from *The Prelude* come from William Wordsworth, *The Prelude, or Growth of a Poet's Mind*, edited by Ernest de Sélincourt, revised by Helen Darbishire (Oxford: Clarendon Press, 1959).

177 "mazy as a river": Geoffrey Hartman, *Wordsworth's Poetry, 1787–1814* (New Haven, Conn.: Yale University Press, 1964), p. 208.

178 "the deep-rooted folk memory": Thompson, *Making of the English Working Class*, p. 357.

179 "the cocks and hens": All quotes from *Adam Bede* come from George Eliot, *Adam Bede* (New York: Harper & Brothers, 1860), pp. 157–75.

179 "all the poetry in which": George Eliot to Sara Sophia Hennell, June 4, 1848, in *The George Eliot Letters*, vol. 1, *1836–1851*, edited by Gordon S. Haight (New Haven, Conn.: Yale University Press, 1954), pp. 263–64.

180 "the old duality of life": All quotes from *The Rainbow* come from D. H. Lawrence, *The Rainbow* (New York: B. W. Heubsch, 1921), chaps. 10 and 11.

185 "And I will make thy seed": Genesis 13:16.

PART SEVEN REMEMBERING THE SABBATH

188 "with Sunday school": Alexis McCrossen, *Holy Day, Holiday: The American Sunday* (Ithaca, N.Y.: Cornell University Press, 2002), p. 138.

189 "freedom from all slavery": G. Stanley Hall, "Sunday Observance," *Pedagogical Seminary* 15 (1908): 221.

191 "reasonable line of demarcation": *McGowan et al. v. Maryland*, 366 U.S. 420 (1961).

192 The first five-day workweek: McCrossen, *Holy Day*, p. 150.

194 One legal scholar: Lesley Lawrence-Hammer, "Red, White, but Mostly

Blue: The Validity of Modern Sunday Closing Laws Under the Establishment Clause," *Vanderbilt Law Review* 60, no. 1273 (May 2007).

195   "The mobile telephone relaxes": Richard Ling, *The Mobile Connection: The Cell Phone's Impact on Society* (San Francisco: Morgan Kaufmann, 2004), p. 74.

197   "Face-to-face social interaction": Randall Collins, *Interaction Ritual Chains* (Princeton, N.J.: Princeton University Press, 2004), p. 78.

198   "The Soviet authorities": Eviatar Zerubavel, *The Seven Day Circle: The History and Meaning of the Week* (Chicago: University of Chicago Press, 1989), pp. 35–43.

199   "the enormous flywheel": William James, *The Principles of Psychology,* vol. 1 (New York: Henry Holt, 1890), p. 121.

200   "When we are learning": Ibid., pp. 112–13.

200   The biologist Eric R. Kandel: Kandel, *In Search of Memory: The Emergence of a New Science of Mind* (New York: W. W. Norton, 2006.)

201   "The mere fact": Max Weber, *Economy and Society: An Outline of Interpretive Sociology,* edited by Guenther Roth and Claus Wittich, translated by Ephraim Fischoff and others (Berkeley: University of California Press, 1978), p. 326.

201   "Processing fluency": Christian Unkelbach, "Reversing the Truth Effect: Learning the Interpretation of Processing Fluency in Judgments of Truth," *Journal of Experimental Psychology: Learning, Memory, and Cognition* 33, no. 1 (2007): 219–30.

201   "We do and we hear": Exodus 24:7.

202   "Leisure is a form of silence": Josef Pieper, quoted in Al Gini, *The Importance of Being Lazy: In Praise of Play, Leisure, and Vacations* (London: Routledge, 2003), pp. 35–36.

202   In 1962: Sebastian de Grazia, *Of Time, Work, and Leisure* (New York: Twentieth-Century Fund, 1962).

203   "Much as the modern-day": David M. Levy, "More, Faster, Better: Governance in an Age of Overload, Busyness, and Speed," in *First Monday,* special issue, no. 7 "Command Lines: The Emergence of Governance in Global Cyberspace," 2006), http://firstmonday.org/htbin/cgiwrap/bin/ojs/index.php/fm/article/view/1618/1533.

204   "relaxation and self-reflection": Jack Wertheimer, ed., *Jews in the Center: Conservative Synagogues and Their Members* (New Brunswick, N.J.: Rutgers University Press, 2000), p. 314.

204   "I love technology": Jill Serjeant, "Taking a Sabbatical from the Internet: Tech Geeks Vow to Wrestle Back Control of Their Lives if Only for a Day," *The Toronto Star,* May 22, 2008.

205   "a mistrust of the pleasures": Michel Foucault, *The History of Sexuality:*

The Care of the Self, translated by Robert Hurley (New York: Vintage, 1990), p. 39. Much of the following comes from this volume, particularly pp. 37–71.

207 Two out of three countries: Stephen Sweet and Peter Meiksins, *Changing Contours of Work: Jobs and Opportunities in the New Economy* (Thousand Oaks, Calif.: Pine Forge Press, 2008), pp. 147–50.

208 "disputes at the boundary of time": Todd D. Rakoff, *A Time for Every Purpose: Law and the Balance of Life* (Cambridge: Harvard University Press, 2002), p. 143.

209 "cultural blindness": Ibid.

212 "Leopards break into": Franz Kafka, *Parables and Paradoxes,* in German and English, edited by Nahum H. Glatzer (New York: Schocken Books, 1961 [1935]).

214 "a repetition and a commemoration": Sigmund Freud, *Totem and Taboo,* translated by A. A. Brill (New York: Random House, 1946), p. 183.

214 "When I was a young man": Sigmund Freud, *The Interpretation of Dreams,* translated by Joyce Crick (Oxford: Oxford University Press, 1999), p. 165.

INDEX

THE
SABBATH
WORLD

Judith Shulevitz

A Reader's Guide

1. Judith Shulevitz says, "The Sabbath does something, and what it does is remarkable" (p. 37). What does the Sabbath do? Do you agree that what it does is remarkable, or do you think all rituals performed by an entire community accomplish more or less the same thing? Do you think the Sabbath could do something remarkable for you or your family?

2. Shulevitz argues that the Sabbath was probably taken over from a Babylonian custom involving the *ume lemnuti,* the evil or inauspicious days, when neither the king nor the priest were allowed to work for fear that they might do harm to their communities. The Fourth Commandment, however ("Remember the Sabbath day and keep it holy"), says nothing about kings or priests. It gives the commandment to you, your household, your servants, your animals, and the stranger at your gate. What's the difference between the Babylonian custom and the commandment? What does the Jewish Sabbath tell us about the people who created it?

3. Why do some people see the Sabbath as having environmental implications? Why do observant Jews refuse to use tools on the Sabbath? What could you do to achieve the same end, even if you don't follow Jewish law?

4. The Sabbath crops up a lot in the Book of Mark—indeed, throughout the Gospels. Jesus preaches on the Sabbath and heals on the Sabbath; Jesus's Sabbath-breaking infuriates the Pharisees so much that they step outside the synagogue and start plotting against him. Shulevitz says that performing miraculous acts on the Sabbath is a way for the Jesus of the Gospels to make a point about time. What's Jesus's point? Did the early Christians believe that Christ's arrival on earth changed the very nature of time? What's the difference between Jewish time and Christian time, according to Shulevitz? Does this explain, in your opinion, the difference between Jews and Christians in their approach to Sabbath-keeping today?

5. The American Puritan Sabbath is notorious for being strict and joyless. But Shulevitz thinks the Puritans found it joyous because it allowed them to re-enact their vision of life in Biblical times. Can you imagine finding the Puritans' Sabbath appealing? Would you like the quiet and hate the discipline, or would you welcome the discipline but secretly chafe at the boredom?

6. Why did America's extensive Sunday-closing laws eventually disappear? Do you think that that was a good thing or a bad thing? How has modern technology changed our sense of time? Does the prevalence of cell phones make it easier or harder to keep the Sabbath?

7. Shulevitz dwells at length on her own feelings of ambivalence toward the Sabbath. Why is she so conflicted about the Sabbath? Do you share her ambivalence, or do you feel wholeheartedly either for or against the Sabbath?

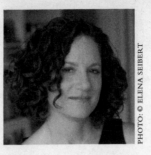

PHOTO: © ELENA SEIBERT

JUDITH SHULEVITZ is a cultural critic and magazine editor who helped to start both *Slate* and *Lingua Franca,* which won a National Magazine Award for General Excellence under her co-editorship. She has been a columnist for *Slate* and *The New York Times Book Review,* and is now contributing editor at *The New Republic.* She lives in New York City.